T0407171

Engineering Approaches to Mechanical and Robotic Design for Minimally Invasive Surgery (MIS)

THE KLUWER INTERNATIONAL SERIES IN ENGINEERING AND COMPUTER SCIENCE

ROBOTICS: VISION, MANIPULATION AND SENSORS

Consulting Editor

Takeo Kanade

Other books in the series:

ROBOT FORCE CONTROL
B. Siciliano, L. Villani
ISBN: 0-7923-7733-8
DESIGN BY COMPOSITION FOR RAPID PROTOTYPING
M. Binnard
ISBN: 0-7923-8657-4
TETROBOT: A Modular Approach to Reconfigurable Parallel Robotics
G.J. Hamlin, A.C. Sanderson
ISBN: 0-7923-8025-8
INTELLIGENT UNMANNED GROUND VEHICLES: Autonomous Navigation Research at Carnegie Mellon
M. Hebert, C. Thorpe, A. Stentz
ISBN: 0-7923-9833-5
INTERLEAVING PLANNING AND EXECUTION FOR AUTONOMOUS ROBOTS
Illah Reza Nourbakhsh
ISBN: 0-7923-9828-9
GENETIC LEARNING FOR ADAPTIVE IMAGE SEGMENTATION
Bir Bhanu, Sungkee Lee
ISBN: 0-7923-9491-7
SPACE-SCALE THEORY IN EARLY VISION
Tony Lindeberg
ISBN 0-7923-9418
NEURAL NETWORK PERCEPTION FOR MOBILE ROBOT GUIDANCE
Dean A. Pomerleau
ISBN: 0-7923-9373-2
DIRECTED SONAR SENSING FOR MOBILE ROBOT NAVIGATION
John J. Leonard, Hugh F. Durrant-Whyte
ISBN: 0-7923-9242-6
A GENERAL MODEL OF LEGGED LOCOMOTION ON NATURAL TERRAINE
David J.Manko
ISBN: 0-7923-9247-7
INTELLIGENT ROBOTIC SYSTEMS: THEORY, DESIGN AND APPLICATIONS
K. Valavanis, G. Saridis
ISBN: 0-7923-9250-7
QUALITATIVE MOTION UNDERSTANDING
W. Burger, B. Bhanu
ISBN: 0-7923-9251-5
NONHOLONOMIC MOTION PLANNING
Zexiang Li, J.F. Canny
ISBN: 0-7923-9275-2

ENGINEERING APPROACHES TO MECHANICAL AND ROBOTIC DESIGN FOR MINIMALLY INVASIVE SURGERY (MIS)

ALI FARAZ
Experimental Robotics Laboratory (ERL)
School of Engineering Science
Simon Fraser University
Burnaby, British Columbia
CANADA

SHAHRAM PAYANDEH
Experimental Robotics Laboratory (ERL)
School of Engineering Science
Simon Fraser University
Burnaby, British Columbia
CANADA

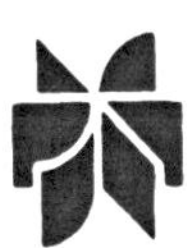

Kluwer Academic Publishers
Boston/Dordrecht/London

Distributors for North, Central and South America:
Kluwer Academic Publishers
101 Philip Drive
Assinippi Park
Norwell, Massachusetts 02061 USA
Telephone (781) 871-6600
Fax (781) 871-6528
E-Mail <kluwer@wkap.com>

Distributors for all other countries:
Kluwer Academic Publishers Group
Distribution Centre
Post Office Box 322
3300 AH Dordrecht, THE NETHERLANDS
Telephone 31 78 6392 392
Fax 31 78 6546 474
E-Mail <orderdept@wkap.nl>

Electronic Services <http://www.wkap.nl>

Library of Congress Cataloging-in-Publication Data

Faraz, Ali.
Engineering approaches to mechanical and robotic design for minimally invasive surgeries (MIS) / Ali Faraz, Shahram Payandeh.
p. cm. -- (Kluwer international series in engineering and computer science)
Includes index.
ISBN 0-7923-7792-3
1. Surgical instruments and apparatus--Design and construction. 2. Endoscopic surgery. 3. Robotics in medicine. 4. Biomedical engineering. I. Payandeh, Shahram, 1957- II. Title. III. Series.

RD71.F36 2000
610'.28--dc21

00-020445

Printed on acid-free paper.

Printed in the United States of America

Contents

List of Figures

List of Tables

Preface

Within the past twenty years, the field of robotics has been finding many areas of applications ranging from space to underwater explorations. One of these areas which is slowly gaining popularity among the users group is the notion of service robotics. This book is an investigation and exploration of engineering principles in the design and development of mechanisms and robotic devices that can be used in the field of surgery. Specifically the results of this book can be used for designing tools for class of Minimally Invasive Surgery (MIS).

Generally, Minimal Invasive Surgery (MIS), e.g. laparoscopic surgery, is performed by using long surgical tools, that are inserted through small incisions at the ports of entry to the body (e.g. abdominal wall) for reaching the surgical site. The main drawback of current designs of endoscopic tools is that they are not able to *extend* all the movements and sensory capabilities of the surgeon's hand to the surgical site. By improving surgical procedures, training, and more practice, it is possible for surgeons to reduce completion time for each task and increase their level of skill. However, even in the best cases the level of performance of a surgeon in Minimally Invasive Surgery is still a fraction of the conventional surgery. Any dramatically improvement is usually driven by introduction of new tools or systems that in turn bring totally new procedures and set of skills. This book studies problems associated with MIS (e.g. laparoscopic surgery), and related tools, which leads to new designs, prototypes, and developments of new tools and systems that can improve the surgical performance.

From an engineering stand point this book addresses problems associated with such surgery and casts them based on engineering design principles. The approach taken here can be followed for developing any similar mechanisms, robotic device or man/machine systems which are applied to confined and restricted work-volumes. In addition, the approach taken in this book is very general, so it can be used in the mechanical design, optimal design, mechatronics systems and robot trajectory planning and control.

This book studies some of the problems associated with laparoscopic surgery, and its primary objectives and motivations are classified in two major categories : a) *dexterity enhancement*, and b) *remote manipulation*. The first class based on *dexterity enhancement* leads us to new designs, prototypes, and developments that can improve the surgical performance, in the themes outlined below.

Adding Dexterity through the Design of Laparoscopic Stand: Positioning of tools, and keeping them in a fixed configuration is a routine task in laparoscopy. This is usually done at the cost of having an assistant surgeon in the operating room, which can also cause crowding of the room. An alternative would be the use of a positioning stand. This patented design provides a resting frame for the surgeon as well as a rigid base for the end-joints to be moved and locked in a much more controlled manner.

Adding Dexterity by using Flexible Stem Graspers: The present rigid-stem laparoscopic tools provide only 4 degrees of freedom and lack 2 rotational movements at the surgical site. The challenge and difficulty lies in creation of rotary joints on a stem, with only 10 mm diameter, which have to be actuated inside the body. There are three basic designs that are studied. The first one is a single-joint design based on a 4 bar-link actuation mechanism, the second design is a multi-revolute joint design which is actuated by screw mechanisms, and the last one is a multi-spherical joint design actuated by tendon-like wires.

Adding Dexterity through the application of Semi-Automatic Devices: One of the most difficult tasks in laparoscopy is the suturing task. The new patented design allows the task to be performed semi-automatically faster and easier. It comprises a needle with a circular arc shape, that is moved in a circular path. The movement is provided manually by continuous motion of one finger, and the surgeon has control over the needle in the circular path both in terms of its position and direction of movement. The external diameter of prototyped model is 33 mm, which is further miniaturized to 12 mm diameter for laparoscopic applications.

The second class of designs is related to developments which increase the ability of the surgeon in the *remote manipulation* of the surgical tissue.

Grasper with force reflection: In laparoscopic graspers, the grasping force is sensed poorly at the hand of the surgeon. This is mostly due to friction, backlash and stiffness of all the intermediate mechanical linkages. The design and development of a grasper with force reflection is presented by using a *tunable spring* design. Experimental results have shown the practicality of such design concept.

Robotic Extenders for Laparoscopy: The direct hand control of laparoscopic tools through incision points is unnatural, remote, and physically demanding for the surgeon. Improvements in surgical dexterity, comparable to the level of open surgery, are studied through the application of various robotic extenders. The proposed robotic extenders can be used either as automated positioners(e.g. for changing the angle of laparoscopic tools to a desired orientation), or as the slave arm in tele-operation systems.

Acknowledgments

The authors are grateful for the financial support of the Institute for Robotics and Intelligent Systems (IRIS) which is part of the Canadian Networks of Centers of Excellence.

The assistance of the Mechanical Instrumentation Workshop of Simon Fraser University for developing the prototypes of this book is greatly appreciated.

The experimental results and feed-backs are obtained at the Jack Bell Medical Research Center in Vancouver British Columbia and specially from Alex Nagy (MD), were fundamental to keep this research on the right track.

Assistance of our colleagues Andon Salvarinov and William Li for electronic implementation and system integration of the prototypes are greatly appreciated.

This book is dedicated
to our families.

Chapter 1

INTRODUCTION

Since 1990, the field of *Minimally Invasive Surgery* (MIS) has experienced a period of rapid developments as an alternative to the conventional open surgery[5]. In this method (MIS), the monitoring endoscope and surgical instruments are fed through small incision points into the body. Historically, the application of endoscopes for visual examination of internal organs, such as colonoscopy, has a long history which dates back several centuries[36]. However, MIS (also known as *endosurgery*) evolved from the traditional endoscopy by using other surgical equipments in conjunction with the endoscope to not only examine, but also to perform surgical operations on different parts of the body. This has resulted in the emergence of many fields within the endoscopic surgery, such as *arthroscopy, angioscopy*, and *laparoscopy* (Table 1.1).

The field of laparoscopy is related only to operations performed on the abdominal part of the body which are (or are becoming) the preferred approach by general surgeons for many procedures. For example, laparoscopic cholecystectomy is now the treatment of choice in all patients with symptomatic gallstone disease who in the recent past would have been offered open cholecystectomy (the first successful laparoscopic cholecystectomy was performed by Mouret in Lyons, France, in 1987 [55]).

This shift from open surgery to MIS (e.g. laparoscopy) is mainly due to the following reasons:

- Shorter recovery time
- Lower risk of infection
- Less pain/ trauma for the patient
- Reduction in hospital stay/cost

Table 1.1. Some of the fields of endoscopic surgery, and laparoscopic procedures.

Field	Procedure	Description
Colonoscopy		Examination and tumor identification in rectum and colon
Arthroscopy		Examination and repair of skeletal or joint disorders
Angioscopy		Examination and un-clogging of blood vessels
Laparoscopy		Endoscopic surgery performed on abdominal organs
	Cholecystectomy	Gall bladder removal
	Inguinal hernia repair	Repair of hernia
	Appendectomy	Removal of vermiform appendix
	Colectomy	Removal of part or all of the colon

On the other hand, the percentage of cases in laparoscopic surgery which have lead to complications, and mortality are in the reasonable low ranges of 4-5%, and 0.1% respectively[5][62].

1. TYPICAL SET-UP FOR LAPAROSCOPIC SURGERY

There are several possible arrangements for any laparoscopic procedure[66], however the set-up shown in Fig. 1.1 can be considered as a typical arrangement used for many different procedures[55]. In the set-up, the surgeon stands on the side of the patient while camera holder is on his/her left, and the chief assistant and the nurse standing on the opposite side of the bed. There are usually one or two monitors placed on mobile stands at eye level, so everyone has a clear view of the surgical site(Fig. 1.1) where the dissected organ is located. The light source, the camera control box, the insufflator, and the suction/irrigation systems are placed on the lower racks of the monitors stands for clear view and monitoring during the operation.

The arrangement in the operating room described above, considered as the *external* set-up(Fig.1.1), is greatly influenced and dictated by the *internal* set-up at the surgical site(Fig.1.2) for each specific procedure [36]. Usually, in addition to the single incision point for the laparoscope, at least two or more incision points are made on the abdomen for other surgical tools such as graspers, needle drivers, or scissors (Fig. 1.2). The incision point on the abdomen should be sealed around the surgical tool

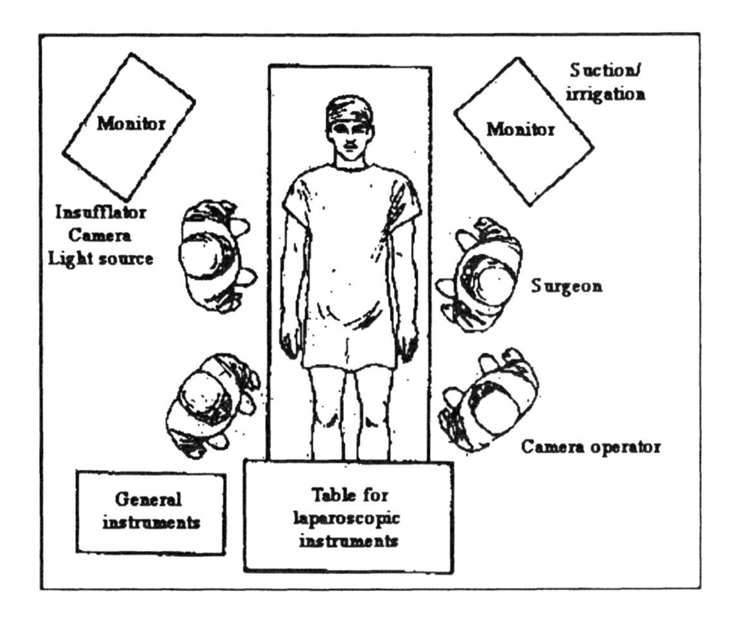

Figure 1.1. The laparoscopic external set-up in the operating room.

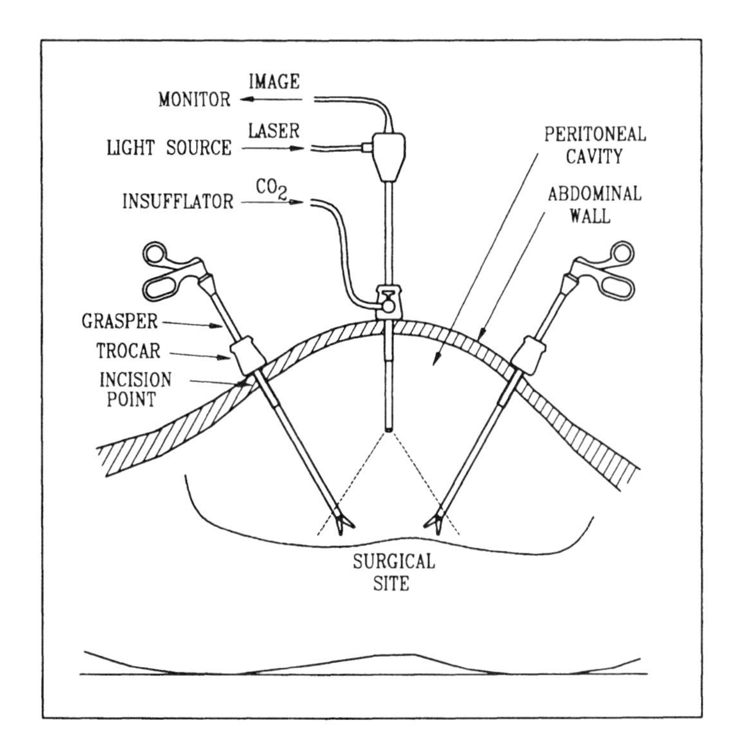

Figure 1.2. The laparoscopic internal set-up on the abdominal region.

with minimal contact friction. This function is provided by the *trocar* at the port of entry. In order to create the work-space at the surgical site, carbon dioxide gas (CO_2) is supplied at a safe pressure level by the insufflator through one of the trocars[36]. The light system consists of a source connected to the laparoscope by a light fiber-optic cable. Visualization of the illuminated peritoneal cavity is achieved by a video camera at the end of the laparoscope that relays the image to video monitors.

Generally, selecting the location of the port of entry for the laparoscope with respect to the other ports of entries(for other tools) is crucial. For example, in cholecystectomy and appendectomy the locations of the incision points are indicated in Fig. 1.3 (where point 1 is for the laparoscope, and points 2, 3, and 4 for other surgical tools/instruments)[13] [68][85]. However, generally in any procedure, the angle between the laparoscope and the surgical tools must not exceed 45°. Otherwise there would be a great decrease in the dexterity of the surgeon due to the loss of hand-eye coordination[87]. To avoid this, the two ports of entry for hand tools(e.g. points 2, and 3, Fig.1.3b) when connected to the port of entry of laparoscope(point 1), forming a triangular configuration, must be proportionally similar and its orientation should correspond to the natural triangle connecting the surgeon's two hands to his eyes location [62].

2. SURGICAL PROBLEMS IN ENDOSURGERY

There are basically three categories of problems in endosurgery: a) Visual problems, b) Movements of hands/tools, and c) Force/tactile sensing, which are described in the following sections:

2.1 VISUAL PROBLEMS

Laparoscopes generally use a video system where the visual information is obtained through a long tube (about 10 mm in diameter and 300 mm in length)[32]. Two types of camera systems, *proximal* and *remote*, are available. In the proximal type, the CCD array is located at the tip of the tube and signals are transmitted through the laparoscope, while in the remote type, the 2D image is transmitted through fiber-optics or lenses to the other end of laparoscope where the CCD camera is located. Both types provide a clear field of view up to 60°. Beside problems associated with capturing a clear image, there are many unsolved problems [32][87] such as:

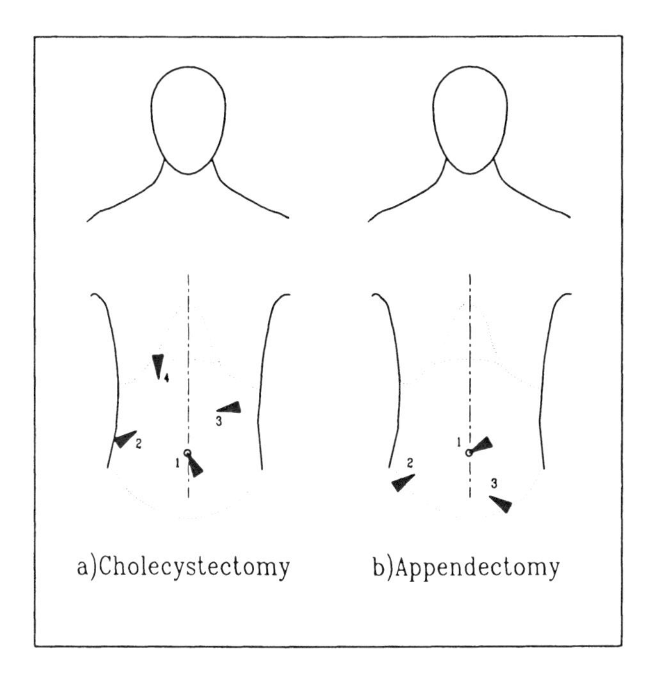

Figure 1.3. The location of ports of entry for cholecystectomy and appendectomy procedures.

- *Lack of stereo-scopic view* : In the case of 2D vision systems, even for simple positioning tasks with endoscopic tools, it takes almost twice the time to perform under direct monocular vision compared to direct binocular vision, and it is even longer (almost 3 times) under the laparoscope viewing condition[60].

- *Limited field of view :* Due to the size limitation of the monitor, as well as the field of view of the laparoscope, the image does not give the natural 150° field of view of human eyes. Therefore the view is not perceived as a natural one, and does not provide a normal working environment for the surgeon to perform the surgical tasks [87][66].

- *Limited resolution :* As a trade-off, the visual resolution could be increased by decreasing the field of view of the laparoscope. However, in this case the resulting resolution is determined by the resolution of the monitor, which is much lower than the resolution of human eyes viewing from a distance[87].

- *Limited contrast and color fidelity.*

There have been some technological advancements in the application of 3D vision systems in the endoscopic surgery. 3D stereo endoscopes available on the market, from quite a few different manufacturers, have improved the depth perception and consequently performance [60]. However, this kind of vision system requires the surgeon to wear special eye-pieces which might not be convenient for some.

On the other hand, there are some practical considerations that if taken into account, can improve the performance greatly. *a) Position of the monitor:* The distance of the monitor from the surgeon should be arranged so that the angle of view of monitor is the same as the angular field of view of the laparoscope. *b) Position and orientation of the laparoscope:* It is important to adjust the axial position of the laparoscope for the optimum resolution/magnification. On the other hand it is even more important to select the proper incision points for the laparoscope to give the natural viewing angle of the surgical site and surgical tools(see Sec.1, Fig.1.3). Also, to have the proper viewing orientation on the monitor, the laparoscope should be able to rotate around its central axis, so that the general orientation of the vision on the monitor would be the same as the vertical orientation of the surgeon.

2.2 MOVEMENTS OF HANDS/TOOLS

The requirement to perform the operation through small incisions limits the available surgical movements, as well as the degrees of freedom [66]. In general, the incision point and the trocar act as a spherical joint on the abdominal wall that allows only three rotational movements(around axes X, Y, and Z, Fig.1.4) and one axial movement(along Z axis) at the joint[32]. The inherent problems associated with this spherical configuration of movements are :

- *Reverse Motion:* The pivoting of the tool around the incision point causes the effect of reverse motion at the handle. This means for example when tools tip should move to the right, the surgeon must move his/her hand to the left. It is a matter of long training and practice to get used to this unnatural reverse motions.

- *Movements Scaling:* The *ratio* of the movement of the tool(ΔT) to the movement of the hand (ΔH) is determined by the distance of the incision point to the surgical site (i.e. $L1$ the length of tool inside the body, Fig. 1.4) divided by the outside length of the tool (i.e. $L2$) [32].

$$\frac{\Delta T}{\Delta H} = \frac{L1}{L2} \tag{1.1}$$

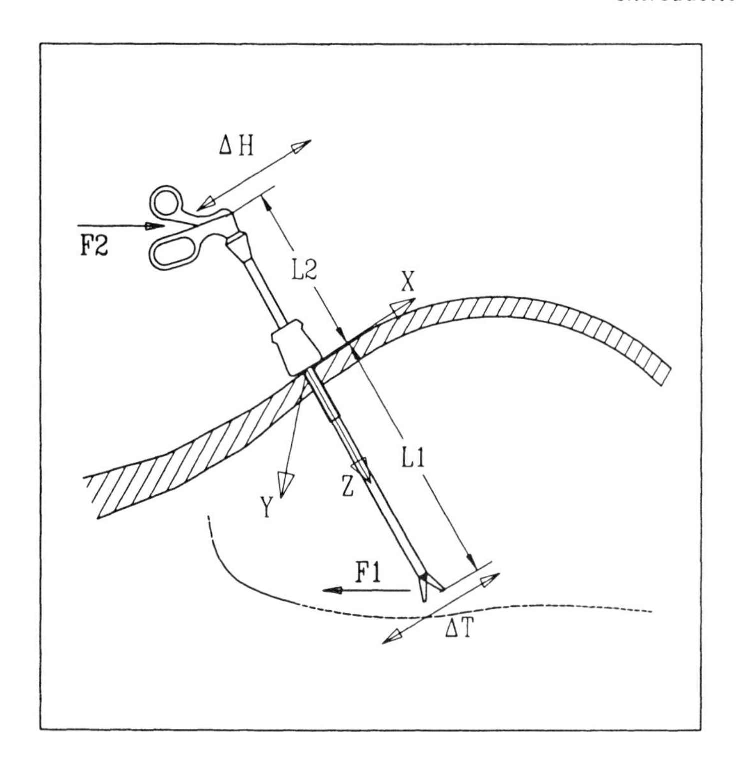

Figure 1.4. The movement of laparoscopic grasper around the incision point.

Therefore, depending how much of the tool is inside the body, the scaling factor of movements varies. This causes the surgeon to be constantly in a state of uncertainty about the amount of required movements, and as a result often makes mistakes in precise movements.

- *Fixed Orientation:* Basically, for the proper manipulation of the tissue and the suturing needle, 3 degrees of rotational movement are required at the surgical site (in addition to the available 3 DOF for the positioning). With the current design of tools with a rigid stem, only one rotational movement around the axis of the stem is possible. Especially in the case of complicated tasks (e.g. suturing), the importance of the tool's orientation at the surgical site is prominent. For example, under identical experimental conditions(for both the direct binocular vision and the indirect endoscopic vision[87]), suturing a square knot with laparoscopic tools took almost twice as long as hand tools used in open surgery.

2.3 FORCE/TACTILE SENSING

Force sensing at the tip of a surgical tool is an important feature for the more efficient and safer performance of tasks such as: cutting, testing, moving, and suturing tissues. Due to the length of laparoscopic tools, and the presence of friction and backlash in its linkages, forces are transmitted very poorly to the hand[66][67] [82][83]. In addition, the lever effect of the tool around the incision point changes the magnitude and the direction of these forces ($F2/F1 = L1/L2$, Fig. 1.4).

Also the tactile sensing is important for sensing the surface texture, and detecting small movements such as pulses in an artery. In laparoscopic tools all of the information is lost and only the grasping force of the tool is sensed to some extent by the surgeon. Of course even in this case, its magnitude and stiffness is altered by all the intermediate mechanical linkages[22][82][83][90].

3. RESEARCH OBJECTIVES

The scope of problems mentioned in the previous section provides the motivation for research in various fields such as:

1. Mechanism and machine design
2. Man-machine haptic interface
3. Robotics and tele-operation
4. New sensor and actuator technologies
5. Optics and endoscopic vision systems
6. Task analysis(time and motion studies) of laparoscopic procedures

However, the focus of this book is within the first three themes which address some of the issues and problems described in Sec.2.2 (movements of hands/tools), and Sec.2.3(force sensing).

Within the above-mentioned research themes, the primary objectives and motivations of this book are classified in two major categories: a) *dexterity enhancement*, and b) *remote manipulation*, which are described in the following sections.

3.1 DEXTERITY ENHANCEMENT

Even with extensive training and practice, the dexterity of the surgeon in laparoscopic surgery is a fraction of that in open surgery when using the current design of tools and systems[87]. This could be improved by enhancing the current design of surgical tools, and techniques, as well as introducing new designs.

Generally, equipments used in the laparoscopic surgery can be divided into two categories of : *I) external* equipment (which provides support for the surgeon without being directly used inside the body at the surgical site, e.g. the bed, tables, anaesthetic machine, etc.), and *II) internal* instruments (which are used or applied inside the peritoneal cavity, e.g. laparoscope, grasper, needle, etc.). In this regard, new tools/devices for dexterity enhancement can be developed with *external* or *internal* functionality types as follows:

- **Adding External Dexterity Through the Design of Laparoscopic Stand**

  In order to perform laparoscopic surgery efficiently for a long period of time, there is a need for a proper working environment for the surgeon to perform surgical tasks[23][26] [28]. The laparoscopic positioning stand provides the *external* support which helps the surgeon to perform the tasks with more ease and dexterity(Ch.2).

- **Adding Internal Dexterity by Additional DOF**

  The current design of laparoscopic tools(e.g. graspers, needle drivers, or scissors) with rigid stems allows only 4 DOF inside the abdominal cavity compared to what is available through the human hand in open surgery with more than 36 DOF[66]. In Ch.3, three types of flexible stems [25][32], which can provide at least two additional DOF for the dexterous manipulation of tissues or needles at the surgical site, are discussed and compared.

- **Internal Automated Devices for Set of Tasks**

  Another method of improving the internal dexterity of the surgeon is by developing new devices that can perform a *group* or *set* of motions automatically(e.g. motions which are required in suturing or knotting). Chapter 4 describes the development of a new type of the suturing device which can help the surgeon to perform the suturing and knotting tasks better and faster [24][32].

3.2 REMOTE MANIPULATION

Due to the remote location of the surgical site in the endoscopic (e.g. laparoscopic operation, most of the sensations which are naturally available in an open surgery are eliminated. Hence the control of the motion/force of various manipulating tasks is more difficult to achieve[66]. The following would provide better force reflection and remote manipulating control for the surgeon.

- **Grasper with Force Reflection**

  The sensation of the grasping force is not reflected properly by laparoscopic forceps[82] [83]. Also, the mechanical linkages provide only a fixed ratio of the transmission of the force from the grasper to the hand(and vice versa), which does not provide an adjustable proportional force reflection. In addition, it is not possible for the surgeon to set a certain maximum limit on the grasping force with current laparoscopic graspers when manipulating soft tissues. In Ch.5, the design of a grasper with the force reflection capability is studied and designed[1][22] [27] [33], which can regulate both the force transmission ratio, as well as controlling the maximum limit of grasping force.

- **Robotic Extenders**

  For better manipulation of tissue remotely, or better viewing of the surgical site, robotic end-effectors with advanced mechanisms, actuations, and control can be designed. The robotic extenders can be used either as (e.g. for changing the angle of endoscope's view to a desired orientation), or as the slave arm in tele-operation systems [29] [31][32]. In Ch.6, kinematic models of such robotic extenders are studied for free motion, and constrained motion cases. The constrained motions involve two cases of: a) *fixed orientation*, which the extender moves while its orientation does not change with respect to the base frame, b) *fixed position*, when the orientation of the extender is changed but the position of its end-point remains the same.

The related literature, and current industrial developments in each of the above mentioned systems are reviewed at the beginning of each chapter. Moreover, in each chapter, different steps of design synthesis, simulation, and experimental results, as well as discussions are provided. Finally in Chapter 7, the contributions of the research are reported, and suggestions for future research work are summarized.

4. BOOK OVERVIEW AND CONTRIBUTIONS

- **Laparoscopic Positioning Stand:** With the motivation of creating a supporting environment for the surgeon to perform the laparoscopic surgery with ease and efficiency, the positioning stand as a new passive system has been designed and developed[23][28]. The patented design[26] comprises a novel application of a concentric multi-link spherical joint as the wrist mechanism, as well as modular arms.

- **Flexible Stems:** Three different types of flexible stems have been developed for applications in laparoscopic graspers, needle drivers, retractors, and other tissue manipulators, as well as flexible viewing laparoscopes[32]. The study has also led to a new comparative workspace analysis of flex stems[25], as well as mathematical models for joint friction[30]. The mathematical models allow us to evaluate accurately the level of forces required to move or lock various types of joints(i.e. cylindrical pin joints, or spherical joints).

- **Suturing Device:** a new class of design for suturing devices has been patented[24] and developed, which can improve the performance of the surgeon in completing both the suturing as well as the knotting tasks.

- **Laparoscopic Grasper with Adjustable Haptic Interface:** This is a new approach to the haptic interface of laparoscopic graspers to the hand of surgeon [1][22] [27] [33]. The force transmission ratio from the handle to the grasper, and the maximum grasping force is regulated through a novel application of tunable springs coupled with the linkage mechanism of the grasper through a specially designed controller. An experimental prototype of the haptic grasper has been developed, and its experimental performance has been compared with the related analytical and simulation results.

- **Robotic Manipulators/Extenders:** The design configuration of robotic manipulators for laparoscopy with up to 4 and 6 DOF was studied, and kinematic models of such manipulators in free or constrained motion were also analyzed[29][32].

Chapter 2

PASSIVE ROBOTICS: LAPAROSCOPIC STAND

In laparoscopic surgery, the reverse hand movements and the limited force sensing of the remote surgical site, in conjunction with the indirect vision and the straining body posture of the surgeon, decrease his/her dexterity dramatically compared to open surgery. One possible method of enhancing dexterity is by *external* mechanisms which provides support for surgical tools outside the body.

This has been the motivation for a number of research groups [29][34] [64] [86], as well as industrial companies[Andronic, Canada][Computer Motion Inc., USA][Armstrong Projects Ltd., UK] to design/develop different types of external mechanisms. These attempts could be classified under two main classes:

I) **Passive Tool Positioners :** These are passive mechanical designs consisting of serial multi-link arms, which are moved manually by the surgeon. The revolute or spherical joints of linkages can be locked individually (e.g. by manual locks) or simultaneously (e.g. by pneumatic or hydraulic locks)[2]. The main function of such an arm is simply to hold the surgical tools in its proper position, or to retract the tissue/internal organ. However, the application of this type of tool positioner is limited to "stationary" tools (such as retractors and endoscopes which are normally stationary), rather than "movable" tools (e.g. graspers and needle drivers) which are normally moved during the operation and locked only when needed.

II) **Active Tool Positioners :** In this type, the controlled actuation of the tool positioner could provide many new features such as automatic repositioning of the tool to the previously stored locations (e.g. for changing the angle of laparoscope's view to a previously stored orientation) such as AESOP commercial system by Computer Motion Inc.[14], or controlling the field of the laparoscopic view by the head movement of the surgeon (such as EndoSista commercial system by Armstrong Projects Ltd.[3][34]). However, the application of these actuated tool positioners is also limited to "stationary" tools.

Both types of tool-positioners described above are designed for some specific tasks only (e.g. locking tools, or automated repositioning of the endoscope, etc.), without considering other aspects and requirements of laparoscopy.

In general, every human activity requires a suitable environment to be performed properly. For instance, consider a typical activity such as writing. For writing, not only a pen and paper are needed as the primary tools, but also a table and chair are required to provide the necessary environment and resting frame to perform the task properly and efficiently[47][69]. However at present, this is not the case in laparoscopy. Here, the surgeon has to carry and manipulate several tools while performing the operation. This is also done in an awkward physical posture which lasts for a long time. In this thesis, one objective is to investigate different designs of *external supports* to create the environment by considering surgical needs and requirements, rather than only one or two specific aspects. This has led us to the design of a multi-arm system which provides support, as well as the capability to lock several *movable* tools in various positions (i.e. in general at least three or more tools are required for a typical laparoscopic procedure). In addition, the design should satisfy the following requirements :

1. to avoid obstruction of the workspace of the surgeon,
2. to avoid interference with other surgical tools,
3. to comply with the kinematic constraints of the incision points at the abdominal wall.

The design should also provide a resting frame for the surgeon to manipulate all the surgical tools (either "stationary"or "movable") in a much more controlled manner with higher dexterity. In the following sections, the design steps of such a laparoscopic stand are described through the synthesis of the wrist and arm mechanisms, as well as their integration in a multi-arm passive system.

1. KINEMATIC SYNTHESIS

The overall objective is the optimal design of a passive multi-arm positioning stand, such that each arm serves one of the laparoscopic tools (Fig. 2.1), which consists of:

a) The *end-effector*, or *the wrist*, which holds and orients the surgical tool through the incision point toward the surgical site.

b) The *positioner*, or *the arm*, which positions the wrist/end-effector along with the surgical tool over the incision point.

The positioning of each arm is performed mainly at the *beginning* of each procedure when the incision points are made (e.g. for cholecystectomy and appendectomy see Fig. 1.3)[13][68][85]. While orienting the wrist, along with the tool, is performed *through out* the surgical procedure. These two tasks (i.e. positioning, and orienting tools) are different both in terms of the *type* of movement (i.e. ideally translational for positioning and rotational for orienting tool), as well as their *time* of application during the procedure. Hence an optimum design not only should be able to perform both tasks, but also it should minimize or eliminate any *interdependence* of joints movements between arms and wrists mechanisms. In other words, the orientation of surgical tool is performed through wrist joints, while its positioning would be accomplished through joints on the arm. To achieve this, the positioning mechanism (i.e. the arm) and orienting mechanism (i.e. the wrist) should be kinematically independent or decoupled. In the following sections (Sec.1.1, and 1.2), first the wrist, and then the arm (Sec.2) mechanisms are type and size synthesized. Finally in Sec.3 through 6, different aspects of the system integration and prototyping are described and discussed.

1.1 TYPE SYNTHESIS OF THE WRIST

In laparoscopic surgery, the abdominal wall acts as a kinematic constraint and provides a pivoting point. Through this point the surgeon moves the tool in a conical workspace with the following degrees of freedom :

a) two angular DOF at the incision point in the range of $\pm 70°$ from the vertical axis passing through the incision point,

b) one rotational DOF around the longitudinal axis of tool in the range of $\pm 180°$, and

c) one translational DOF in and out of the abdominal cavity.

This conical workspace is centred on the spherical movement of tool around the incision point, which is the *inherent* and the *primary* kinematic constraint in laparoscopic surgery, and any design of the wrist should be able to provide these required degrees of freedom[62]. As a result, the wrist should have the same DOF as a spherical joint at the

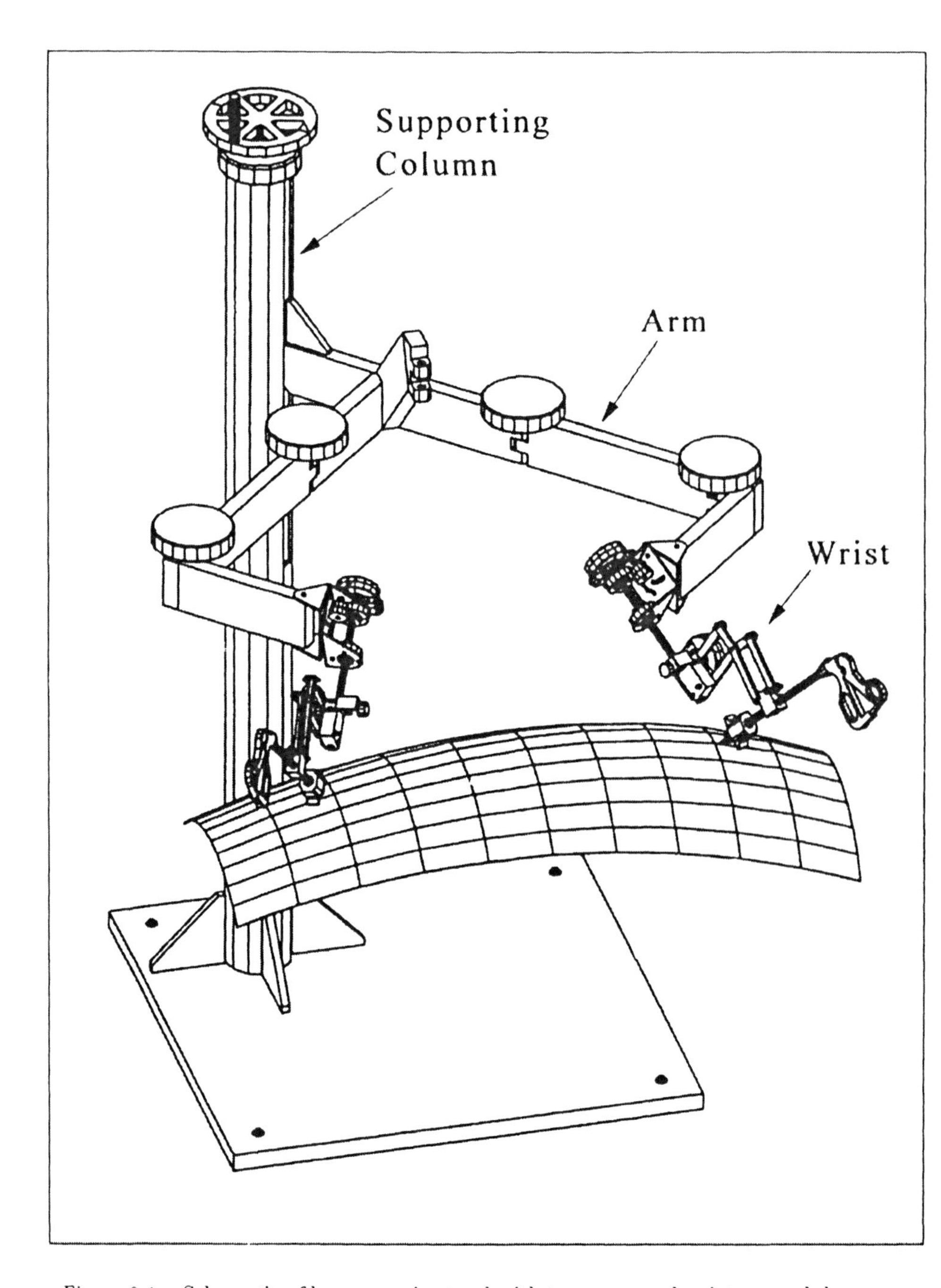

Figure 2.1. Schematic of laparoscopic stand with two arms and wrists over abdomen.

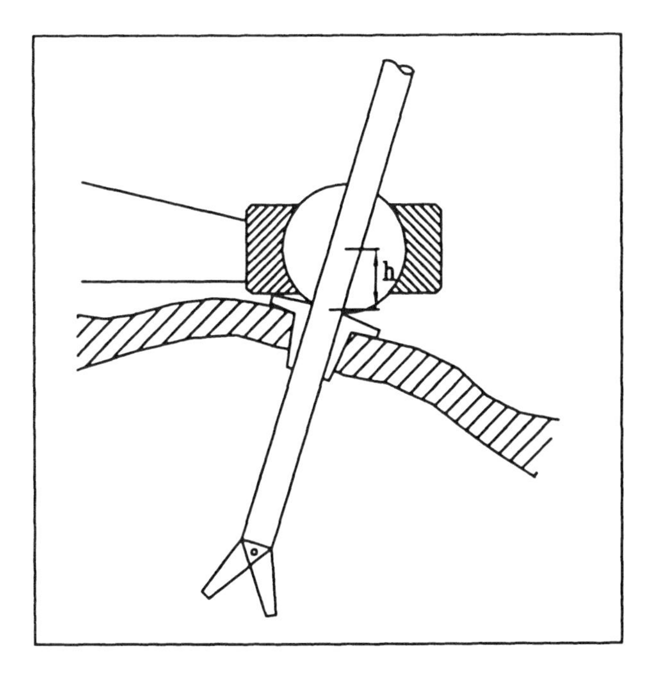

Figure 2.2. The wrist with spherical joint.

incision point, in addition to the linear translational movement through the incision point.

Based on requirements of the design of the wrist, the following type synthesis is limited only to those mechanisms that can provide the required *spherical* movements:

Type I- Spherical joint: This is a spherical joint with socket-ball design. Here, the tool passes through the center of the joint and then through the incision point (Fig. 2.2).

Advantages: 1) it is a compact and light design, 2) it has minimum number of moving parts, and 3) it is simple to design/manufacture.

Disadvantages: 1) it has a low range of movement (much less than the required range of $\pm 70°$), 2) its center of rotation is not at the incision point, but at a distance (**h**, Fig. 2.2). As a result, this design makes it difficult to rotate the tool as a spherical joint about the incision point, and 3) in the case of actuated wrist, it is not very feasible to actuate the socket-ball around the three axes of rotation of the joint.

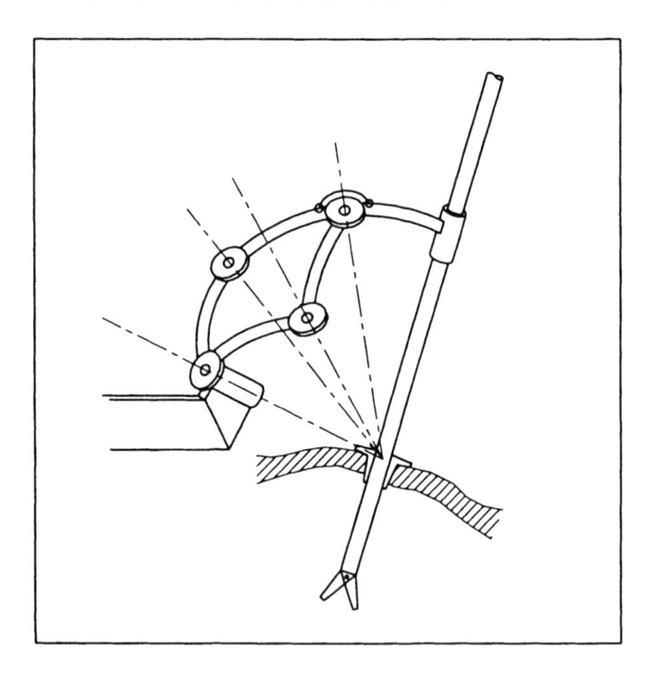

Figure 2.3. The wrist with spherical links mechanism.

Type II- Spherical links: In this design, the linkages are circular arc-shaped with the same radius, where all axes of the joints pass through a central point, i.e. the incision point. To provide two rotational DOF, a spatial five bar spherical linkage could be designed (Fig. 2.3).

Advantages: 1) it provides exactly spherical movement at the incision point, and 2) it has adequate range of angular movements (±70°).

Disadvantages: 1) it does not provide sufficient rigidity, especially when the mechanism is extended to extreme angles, 2) it is prone to clogging and difficult to manipulate due to the clearance of joints, and the misalignment of linkages under the load, and 3) it is bulky, and requires massive joints and linkages in order to increase its rigidity.

Type III- Concentric Multi-link Spherical Joint: This design consists of six linkages and eight rotary joints, which simulates exactly a spherical joint at the point of incision (Fig. 2.4). It can create a large angular range of movement in either directions. The proportions of linkages and locations of joints with respect to one another are in such a way that the orientation of the tool is always toward the fixed point O (i.e. incision point)[43]. Hence, the tool can be made to rotate about the point O around the three perpendicular directions (i.e. X,Y, and Z axes, Fig. 2.4), which is similar to a spherical joint.

Advantages: 1) it can exactly create the spherical movement about the incision point, 2) it has a wide range of angular movement (more than ±70°), and 3) it can be made very compact which does not occupy too much of space (specially in the horizontal plane above the abdominal area) compared to Type II.

Disadvantage: The only disadvantage could be lack of absolute rigidity due to the higher number of joints. To minimize this, special attention should be given to the joints clearances at the stage of detailed design.

In summary, comparing the above three types of wrist mechanisms and considering the disadvantages of each, the concentric multi-link spherical joints has multiple advantages as a better type of wrist end-effector, which is size synthesized in the next section.

1.2 SIZE SYNTHESIS OF THE WRIST

To determine the size of mechanism and its geometry, the following parameters are defined based on Fig. 2.4 :

L_1 is the distance of joints B and E from the incision point (point O) along axes Y and Z respectively.

L_2 is the size of linkages AB, CD, FD, and EG.

L_3 is the distance of EG, and AB from axes Z, and Y respectively.

L_4 is the the size of linkages AC, BD, ED, and FG.

ϕ is the bent angle in the shank of linkages FDB, and CDE at the point D.

The kinematic derivations of the mechanism by Hamlin[43] , lead us to the following equality constraints, which should be satisfied in order for the concentric multi-link spherical joint[43] to function exactly like a spherical joint:

$$\tan\phi = \frac{L_3}{L_1}, \qquad \sin\phi = \frac{L_3}{L_4}$$

From the above equations, it is evident that size L_2 does not play any role in the kinematics functionality of the mechanism. However, it will be shown later that size L_2 is an important parameter in the kinetic analysis of the mechanism. In fact, the magnitudes of quasi-static reaction forces, which can act on all the joints under the influence of an external load, are greatly influenced by size L_2.

To demonstrate this, let us consider the case when joints A and H are locked to prevent the mechanism from any movement (Fig. 2.4). Let external moment M be applied to the linkage GE. In order to find the reaction forces (F_1, and F_2) at joints (A,B,C,E,F,G, and D respectively) to the external load, we can write the equilibrium equations for links

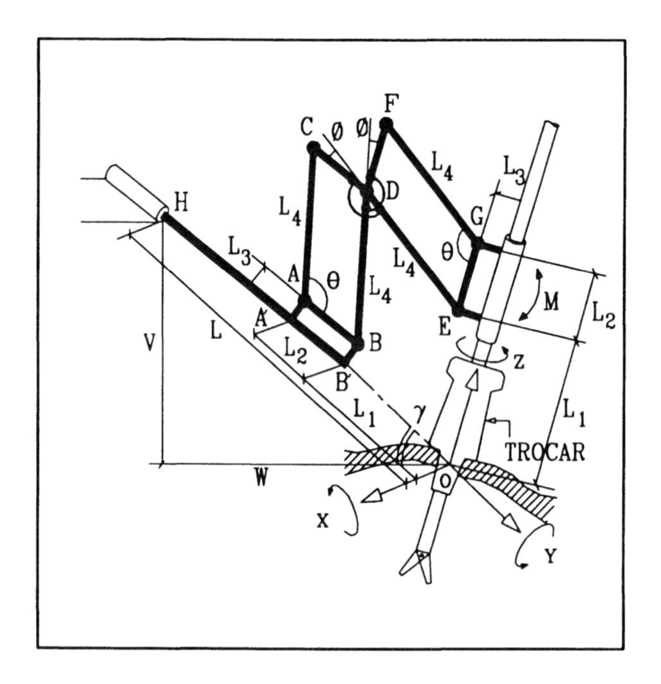

Figure 2.4. The concentric multi-link spherical joint

CDE and FDB, and then solving simultaneously we can obtain:

$$F_1 = \frac{M}{L_2 \sin\theta}, \; F_2 = \frac{M}{L_4 \sin\theta}, \; \text{or} \; \frac{F_1}{F_2} = \frac{L_4}{L_2}$$

The above equations show that forces at the joints F_1 or F_2 approach infinity if either the size of L_2 or L_4 approaches zero. Therefore to avoid extreme forces at joints, we must limit the links ratio $\frac{L_4}{L_2}$. Here, the ratio of 2 is considered as the extreme factor on non-uniformity of reaction forces at different joints in order to proceed with the design, which leads us to the following constraint ratio of linkages:

$$2 \geq \frac{L_4}{L_2} \geq \frac{1}{2} \tag{2.1}$$

Other constraints of the mechanism can be written as:

$$L_1 \geq 80^{mm}, L_3 \geq 20^{mm} \tag{2.2}$$

Where $L_1 \geq 80$ represents the space required for the trocar from point O to E (Fig. 2.4), and $L_3 \geq 20$ represents the expected space requirements of the joints at points A,B,E, and G.

The objective of the following optimization is to minimize the overall size of the wrist mechanism, which could be achieved by various objective functions. One approach would be minimizing the length OH (Fig. 2.4). Since, $OH = OB' + A'B' + A'H$ where, $A'B' = L_2, OB' = L_1$, and to avoid interference between joints C and H when θ approaches 180° we define $A'H > L_4$, hence the minimum value of OH can be defined as:

$$Minimized: OH = L_1 + L_2 + L_4 = L_1 + L_2 + \frac{L_3}{\sin\phi} \equiv L \qquad (2.3)$$

The above objective function is solved numerically subject to the inequality constraints (2.1), and (2.2). The optimal values are obtained to be: $L_1 = 80mm, L_2 = 41mm, L_3 = 20mm, L_4 = 82mm, \phi = 14°$, and $L = 204mm$.

On the other hand, the rotational movement of the tool about X-axis (in CCW direction, Fig. 2.4) is constrained by the inclination of the base shaft HB' (with the angle γ relative to the horizontal plane). In order to maximize the range of the rotational movement of the wrist about X-axis, the angle γ should be minimized. Since length L is already known, to minimize angle γ it is necessary to find the minimum value of distance V, which is the vertical distance of joint H above the abdomen. In general, it is not desirable to get the lower part of the arm any closer than 50 mm to the patient's abdomen (in order to prevent any possible contact between the abdomen and the arm when it is moved in the horizontal plane). As a result, by choosing $V = 50mm$: $\gamma = 14.2°$, and the projection of wrist in the horizontal plane would be: $W = 198mm$.

In the literature, there are other planar designs with some similarity to the wrist mechanism described in this book. For instance, Neisius[64] has proposed and motivated a planar arm mechanism for laparoscopic tele-operation systems. However, the concept is not presented by any specific design. However, Taylor[86] has proposed in detail a parallelogram multi-link system which geometrically is a *special case* of the design described above (when the angle $\phi = 0$). This means linkages FDB, and CDE are straight without the bend, consequently for the mechanism to perform exactly as a spherical joint at the incision point, we must have $L_3 = L_4 \sin\phi = 0$ [43]. This lack of offset L_3 results in spatial interference of joints E and G with the stem of surgical tool (Fig. 2.4).

In addition, both of the above referred planar mechanisms [64][86] have been designed and are intended to be used as a *single positioning arm*. Consequently, these designs (as described by the authors as manipulator arms) can not be considered as wrist mechanisms similar to the proposed design here, which is solely designed as a wrist mechanism, where several of them can be installed on a multi-arm stand to be used in the same limited workspace (Fig. 2.12).

2. SYNTHESIS OF THE POSITIONING ARM

The general requirements for the design of the positioning arm, as a multi-arm passive mechanical system [29][62], are: a) to be a statically balanced mechanism, b) to be easily movable by a hand, c) to be lockable at any location, d) to occupy the least space in the operating area and not to interfere with surgeon's working area, and e) as a multi-arm system, different arms should not interfere with each other.

There are infinite design possibilities for such positioning arms. In some positioning stands and manipulators such as HISAR surgical robot by Funda[37], redundant axes are incorporated in the design of a single arm. This can provide more flexibility and more degrees of freedom to move the arm. On the other hand, any redundant axis can make the system heavier, bulkier and more difficult to manipulate since any additional axis requires stronger and heavier joints/linkages prior to that axis (consequently higher inertia, mass, gravitational and frictional forces). Here the number of axes are kept as few as possible and redundant axes are not included.

To position the end of a manipulator/robot in a three dimensional space, at least 3 degrees of freedom are required. Fig. 2.5 shows different schematic configurations of 3-axis arms with rotary and/or prismatic joints [23][27] [28].

Based on the above stated requirements, there are several mechanisms in Fig. 2.5 that can be considered as good candidates such as No. 12, 13, and 41. No. 12 and 13 are different configurations of three prismatic joints arms (PPP) where X and Z directions of motions are in horizontal plane. Hence, it can be moved easily (since gravitational forces do not have any components in these directions). In addition Y axis could be balanced by the use of counter-balancing mechanisms (e.g. weight pulleys/ pneumatic weight compensators/electric motor balancing systems) or by using self locking lead screw mechanisms. The disadvantage of No.12 and 13 is that prismatic joints can become bulky/massive, and can introduce higher frictional/inertial forces than rotary joints. In addition, both designs are overhead mount, that makes them less attractive from point of view of portability, ease of installation, and maintenance.

The design No.41, on the other hand is a (PRR) SCARA configuration (for Selective Compliant Articulated Robot for Assembly) where the two rotary joints are parallel along the vertical Y axis. The arm is naturally balanced, and can be moved in the horizontal plane, which is parallel to the surface of the operating table. The linkages of the arm can be

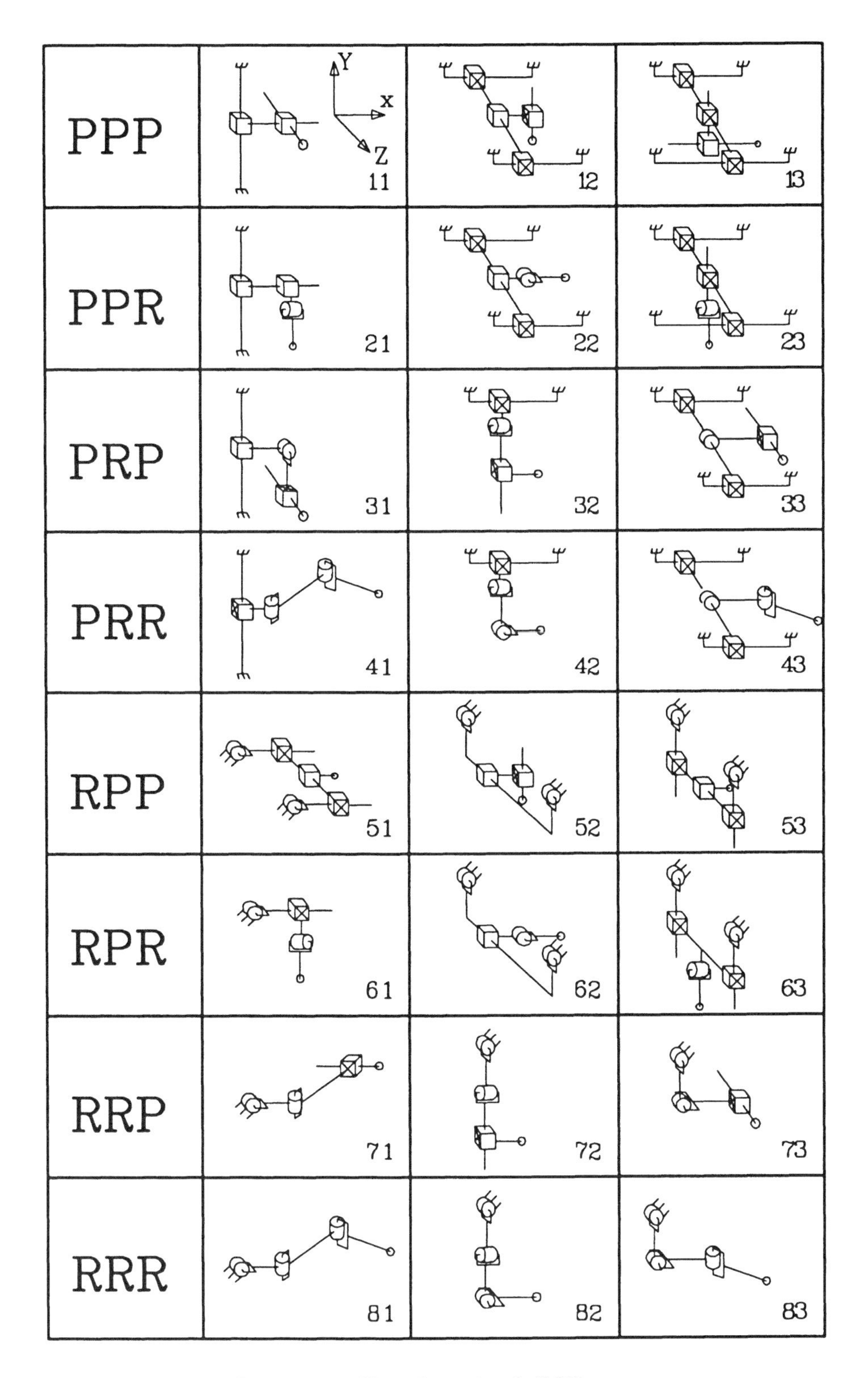

Figure 2.5. The schematic of 3DOF arms.

selected to be short, light, with low friction rotary joints which can be moved manually. All these make the SCARA configuration very attractive for this application.

By selecting SCARA type, the next design issue is related to the workspace that such an arm should reach. In this respect, the maximum operating area over the abdomen with a rectangular shape of 500×350 mm can be considered, which is divided equally in to two areas of 250×350 for each arm (left and right). The surgeon is on the opposite side of the operating table that uses each arm by one of his hands (Fig. 2.12). The surgeon in general should be able to: a) manipulate the arms to the desired positions easily, and b) the dimensions of the arms should allow them to reach their entire work space. To satisfy these requirements, two main topics of *manipulability* and *reachability* of the arms are subsequently studied as parts of the related size synthesis in the next two sections.

2.1 MANIPULABILITY OF THE ARM

The ease of moving the passive arm by the hand of the surgeon depends not only on the friction at each joint, but also on the configuration of the arm, and the size of linkages. The purpose of this section is to study the *manipulability* (which represents the magnitude of manipulating forces at the tip of the arm at a given position in the workspace), and *isotropy* (i.e. the uniformity of the manipulating forces in different directions at a given position in the workspace) of the arm, in order to optimize the size of its linkages, and the range of movements of its joints.

There are several works in the literature that are related to this study with well known concepts such as *manipulability* [53][98], and *isotropy* of manipulating forces [38][50][73]. These concepts have evolved from the definition of *Jacobian* matrix of manipulators[1] (J), the absolute value of the determinant of Jacobian[2] as a measure of manipulability, and the *condition index/number* of the transpose of Jacobian[3]. However, the determinant and the condition index of Jacobian matrix, as measures of *manipulability* and *isotropy* do not represent any physical design parameter. In this section, a new measure of manipulability (i.e. the ratio of the maximum and the minimum manipulating forces at different points of the reachable workspace) is derived as a physical interpretation in-

[1] *Jacobian* matrix (J) is defined as the translator of the velocity state of the joints to the velocity state of the endpoint of the manipulator (i.e. $\dot{X} = J\dot{\theta}$) [4][78].

[2] i.e. $m = |det(J)|$ as the measure of manipulability for non-redundant manipulators [98].

[3] i.e. $C(J^T) = \| J^{-T} \| . \| J^T \|$ as the measure of isotropy[50].

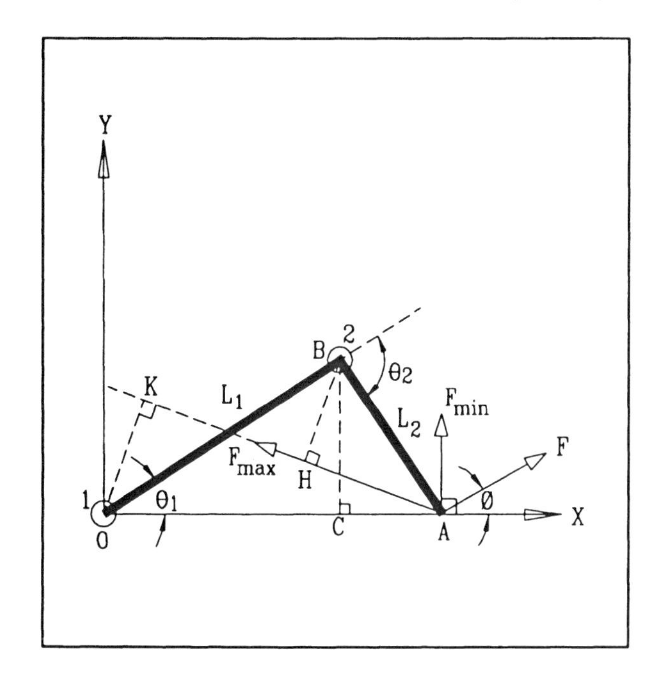

Figure 2.6. Manipulating forces acting on the arm.

stead of the condition index, to the special case of the passive arm with constant frictional torque at the joints.

Based on the notion of singularity, a design of a mechanism loses at least one DOF, when the determinant of Jacobian approaches zero. For two-link mechanism (Fig. 2.6), the Jacobian would be:

$$J = \begin{bmatrix} -L_1 \sin\theta_1 + L_2 \sin(\theta_2 - \theta_1) & L_2 \sin(\theta_2 - \theta_1) \\ L_1 \cos\theta_1 + L_2 \cos(\theta_2 - \theta_1) & L_2 \cos(\theta_2 - \theta_1) \end{bmatrix}$$

and det (J)$=-L_1 L_2 \sin\theta_2 = 0$ when $\theta_2 = 0$, and π.

The manipulability measure (m) for a non-redundant mechanism is the absolute value of determinant Jacobian [53][98]: $m = |det(J)|$. Therefore at $\theta_2 = 0$ and π, the manipulability measure $m = |det(J)|$ would be zero. Also the arm is not manipulated easily due to lack of isotropy as we get close to the singularity points [38][73]. So not only the singularity points (i.e. $\theta_2 = 0, \pi$) must be avoided, but also θ_2 should be limited to the range that the manipulability of the two link system is in an acceptable range. To formulate this, let us consider joint torques relationship: $\tau = J^T F$, where F is the applied hand force acting at the end of arm, at an angle ϕ (Fig. 2.6) :

$$\begin{bmatrix} \tau_1 \\ \tau_2 \end{bmatrix} = [J]^T \begin{bmatrix} F\cos\phi \\ F\sin\phi \end{bmatrix} \tag{2.4}$$

The reaction torque at joints 1 and 2 is basically Coulomb frictional torque, and its maximum limit can be considered to be τ_{max} (so $|\tau_1|$ and $|\tau_2| \leq \tau_{max}$). Hence the minimum force required (in any direction) to move either joint 1 or 2 by producing enough torque (τ_{max}) depends on the normal distance of acting force F, to the joint (Fig. 2.6). To find the minimum and maximum forces to move the arm, the following cases are considered:

I) Case $OA \geq AB$: In this case joint 1 is the first joint to move since it has the longest distance from the manipulating force (i.e. OA, Fig. 2.6). To find the magnitude and direction of the minimum force (F_{min}) that can move joint 1, we have (from Eq. (2.4)):

$$\begin{aligned} \tau_1 = \tau_{max} = \quad & F\cos\phi[-L_1\sin\theta_1 + L_2\sin(\theta_2-\theta_1)] + \\ & F\sin\phi[L_1\cos\theta_1 + L_2\cos(\theta_2-\theta_1)] \end{aligned}$$

Since $L_1 \sin\theta_1 = L_2\sin(\theta_2 - \theta_1)$ (=BC in Fig. 2.6), then the above equation reduces to:

$$F = \frac{\tau_{max}}{\sin\phi[L_1\cos\theta_1 + L_2\cos(\theta_2-\theta_1)]} \tag{2.5}$$

Here F_{min} happens when $\phi = \pm\frac{\pi}{2}$, and by substituting this in(2.5):

$$F_{min} = \frac{\tau_{max}}{L_1\cos\theta_1 + L_2\cos(\theta_2-\theta_1)} \tag{2.6}$$

On the other hand, the maximum force (F_{max}) required to move joint 1 or/and 2 should have the minimum distance from joint 1 and 2 (BH=OK, Fig. 2.6). Any other direction makes the perpendicular distance of force F from either joint 1 or 2 more than BH or OK. Consequently the force required to produce torque τ_{max} around that joint would be less than F_{max}. The angle of F_{max} (i.e. ϕ_{max} where BH=OK, Fig. 2.6) can be obtained analytically by inserting $\tau_1 = \pm\tau_{max}$ and $\tau_2 = \mp\tau_{max}$ in (2.4) to obtain following equations:

$$\begin{aligned} \pm\tau_{max} = \quad & F_{max}\sin\phi_{max}[L_1\cos\theta_1 + L_2\cos(\theta_2-\theta_1)] \\ \mp\tau_{max} = \quad & F_{max}L_2\sin(\theta_2-\theta_1+\phi_{max}) \end{aligned}$$

by dividing the above equations and simplification, we get:

$$\cot\phi_{max} = -2\cot(\theta_2-\theta_1) - \cot(\theta_1) \tag{2.7}$$

Yoshikawa[98] stated the optimum linkage size for manipulability of a two link system is when $L_1 = L_2$, that leads to: $\theta_1 = \theta_2/2$ (Fig. 2.6). By substituting this in (2.7):

$$\cot \phi_{max} = -3\cot(\theta_2/2) \tag{2.8}$$

Also from (2.5):

$$F_{max} = \frac{\tau_{max}}{\sin \phi_{max}[L_1 \cos \theta_1 + L_2 \cos(\theta_2 - \theta_1)]} \tag{2.9}$$

The ratio of (2.9) over (2.6) would be:

$$\frac{F_{max}}{F_{min}} = \frac{1}{\sin \phi_{max}} \tag{2.10}$$

And by substituting (2.8) in (2.10), the ratio of maximum and minimum manipulating forces when $OA \geq AB$ can be obtained as:

$$\frac{F_{max}}{F_{min}} = \sqrt{1 + 9\cot^2(\theta_2/2)} = \frac{\sqrt{2(1+\cos\theta_2)(5+4\cos\theta_2)}}{\sin\theta_2} \tag{2.11}$$

II) Case $OA \leq AB$: In this case joint 2 is the first joint to move. The magnitude and direction of the minimum force that moves joint 2 with torque τ_{max} according to equation (2.4) is: $\tau_2 = \tau_{max} = FL_2 \sin(\theta_2 - \theta_1 + \phi)$, hence:

$$F = \frac{\tau_{max}}{L_2 \sin(\theta_2 - \theta_1 + \phi)} \tag{2.12}$$

And F_{min} happens when $\sin(\theta_2 - \theta_1 + \phi) = 1$:

$$F_{min} = \frac{\tau_{max}}{L_2} \tag{2.13}$$

The magnitude and direction of F_{max} can be established in the same way as the previous case, which also leads to equations (2.8) and (2.9). So the ratio of maximum and minimum forces when $OA \leq AB$, for the case $L_1 = L_2$ and $\theta_1 = \theta_2/2$ would be:

$$\frac{F_{max}}{F_{min}} = \frac{\sqrt{1 + 9\cot^2(\theta_2/2)}}{2\cos(\theta_2/2)} = \frac{\sqrt{5+4\cos\theta_2}}{\sin\theta_2} \tag{2.14}$$

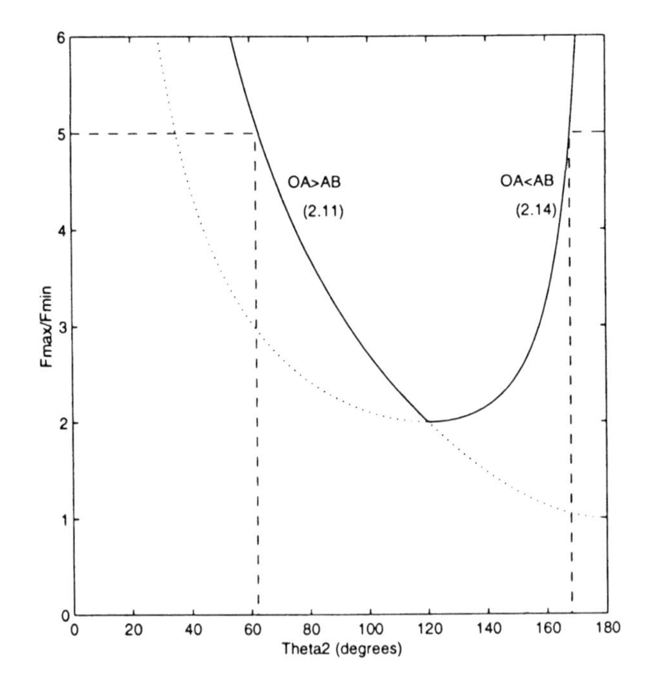

Figure 2.7. F_{max}/F_{min} vs. θ_2

$\frac{F_{max}}{F_{min}}$ as a *new* local measure of manipulability (or isotropy) is plotted against θ_2 in Fig. 2.7, to able the designer to choose the best range of θ_2 that the isotropy of manipulating forces is in the acceptable range. For the design of the positioning arm, let the initial range of the above manipulability measure to be: $5 \geq \frac{F_{max}}{F_{min}} \geq 2$

According to Fig. 2.7, this leads to the following range of θ_2 based on equations (2.11), and (2.14): $168° \geq \theta_2 \geq 60°$.

However, the upper limit of θ_2 should be decreased further to 135°, due to the constraint caused by the requirement for the orientation of the wrist (which is discussed in Sec. 3.). Therefore the final range of θ_2 that would be acceptable for the local manipulability, as well as the wrist orientation would be : $135° \geq \theta_2 \geq 60°$.

2.2 REACHABILITY OPTIMIZATION

The objective of this section is to minimize the arm's size while ensuring it still can reach the entire operating area of $350 \times 250mm$ subject to the manipulation and orientation constraints $135° \geq \theta_2 \geq 60°$.

The variables of this optimization are the arm's base position (a and b, Fig. 2.8), and the size of linkages (L_1 and L_2). For a given position and linkage sizes (i.e. a, b, L_1, and L_2), in order for the the arm (ABC)

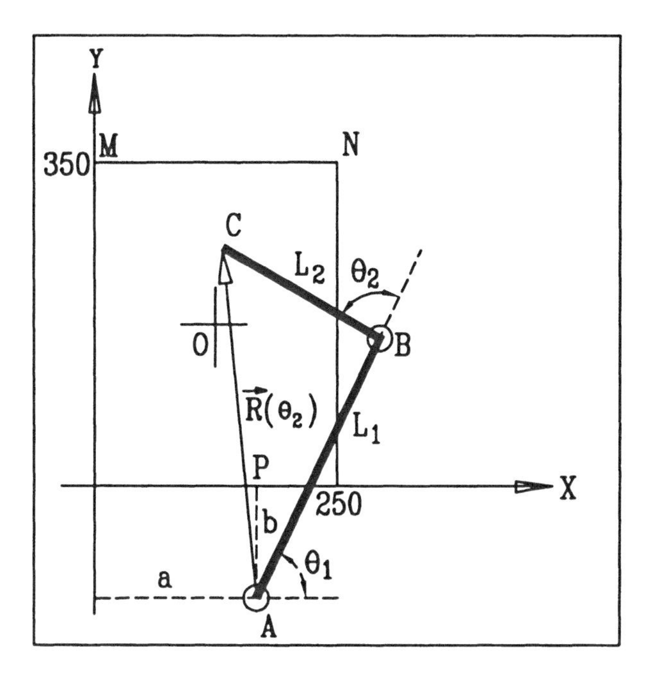

Figure 2.8. The arm's variables (a, b, L_1, and L_2.)

to reach the farthest point (M or N), we need to have:

$$\left|\vec{R}(\theta_2 = 60°)\right| \geq MAX(AMorAN),$$

this leads to :

$$L_1^2 + L_2^2 + L_1 L_2 \geq MAX[a^2 + (b+350)^2, (250-a)^2 + (b+350)^2] \quad (2.15)$$

To reach the nearest point (P):
$\left|\vec{R}(\theta_2 = 135°)\right| \leq AP$, This leads to:

$$L_1^2 + L_2^2 - \sqrt{2} L_1 L_2 \leq b^2 \quad (2.16)$$

These two inequality constraints (2.15), and (2.16) ensures that thearm can reach all the points in its workspace without violating the manipulability constraint $135° \geq \theta_2 \geq 60°$.

The objective function for this optimization is to minimize the overall size of the arm. One way of achieving this is by minimizing the distance of the base point A from the central point of the workspace (i.e. point O, Fig. 2.8). Hence the objective function can be formulated as :

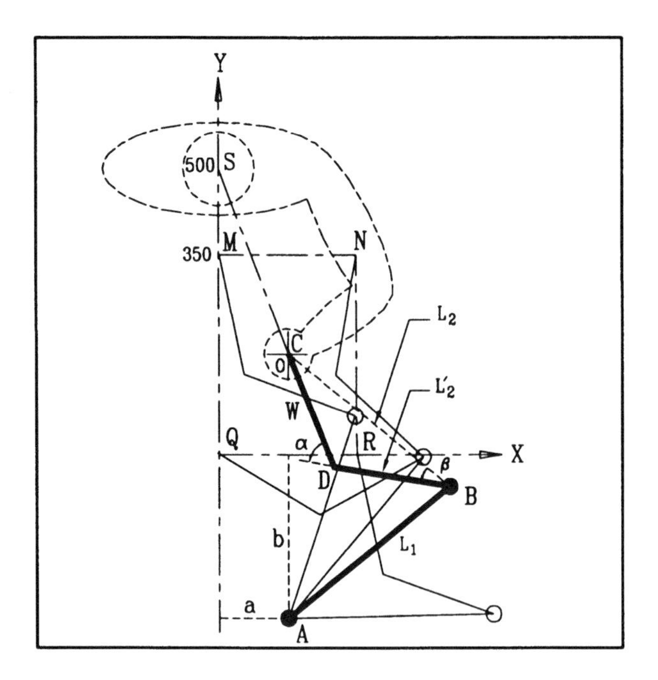

Figure 2.9. The wrist with orientation toward point S.

$$MIN : f(a,b) = AO^2 = (a - 125)^2 + (b + 175)^2 \qquad (2.17)$$

Subject to the inequality constraints (2.15) and (2.16), the results are obtained to be: $a = 125, b = 287, L_1 = L_2 = 375mm$.

3. MULTI-ARMS INTEGRATION

To minimize the obstruction caused by the planar linkage mechanism of the wrist in the operating area of the surgeon, it is desirable to have the orientation of wrist (W) always pointing toward the surgeon at point S (Fig. 2.9). In other words, the wrist mechanism (W) should be configured in such an orientation that it would always be located on the opposite side of surgeon. Here the incision point (C) is considered as the center point in between [23] [28][62].

Ideally joint D could be an actuated joint, so that angle α could be controlled based on the configuration of the arm in such a way that wrist W always points toward the surgeon when point C is moved. Another design could be when joint D is considered as a fixed joint with constant angle α. This design would be satisfactory if the deviation of the orientation of the wrist from its initial orientation (i.e. OS, Fig. 2.9) is in an acceptable range (e.g. $\pm 45°$) for the entire operating workspace.

This could be verified by finding the fixed value of α, β, and L_2' when C is at the center of the operating area while W is pointing toward S (where $x_s = 0$ and $y_s = 500$). Using the optimized values of a, b, L_1, L_2, and W from previous sections, and using basic geometric analysis we can obtain: $\alpha = 58°$, $\beta = 27°$, $L_2' = 230mm$

As shown in Fig. 2.9, the orientation of the wrist does not deviate (from its initial orientation OS) more $\pm 45°$ for extreme points of the operating area (e.g. points M,N,Q, and R). Also wrist W does not interfere with the operating area of the other arm when approaching the symmetrical axis of Y. Therefore for a passive positioning arm, a fixed joint at D at constant angle α could be considered as a suitable type, and also the simplest solution.

Another result of adopting joint D with angle $\alpha = 58°$, is limiting further the rotational range of joint B (i.e. $135° \geq \theta_2 \geq 60°$, Sec.2.1). This is due to the fact that angle DBA should be greater than 15° in order to avoid interference of joint D with link AB. This angle (i.e. $\geq 15°$) added to $\beta = 27°$, would cause angle θ_2 to be limited to the maximum value of 135°. Therefore the final range of θ_2 that satisfies both manipulability, as well as the wrist-orientation would be: $135° \geq \theta_2 \geq 60°$.

4. FEATURES OF MECHANICAL DESIGN

The laparoscopic stand is a passive system whose joints have locking mechanisms. When needed during the operation, it is possible to maintain its configuration in a locked position. For the two joints of each arm (i.e. A, and B, Fig. 2.9), as well as two joints of the wrist (i.e. H, and A, Fig. 2.4), there are different possibilities and types of locking mechanisms. The main requirements for the locking mechanism are :

1. To be compact and light,
2. To be directly mounted on the joint,
3. To have sufficient locking torque, and
4. To provide easy actuation without any contamination.

The locks must resist torques caused by hand forces (up to 50N)[15] exerted by the surgeon. Based on the configuration of the arm and the wrist, this would create maximum torques ($\tau = F.L$) up to 35 and 10 Nm on the joints of arms and wrists respectively. Magnetic commercial breaks for this range of torques are relatively massive, and do not satisfy the first requirement. The hydraulic breaks are very compact and light,

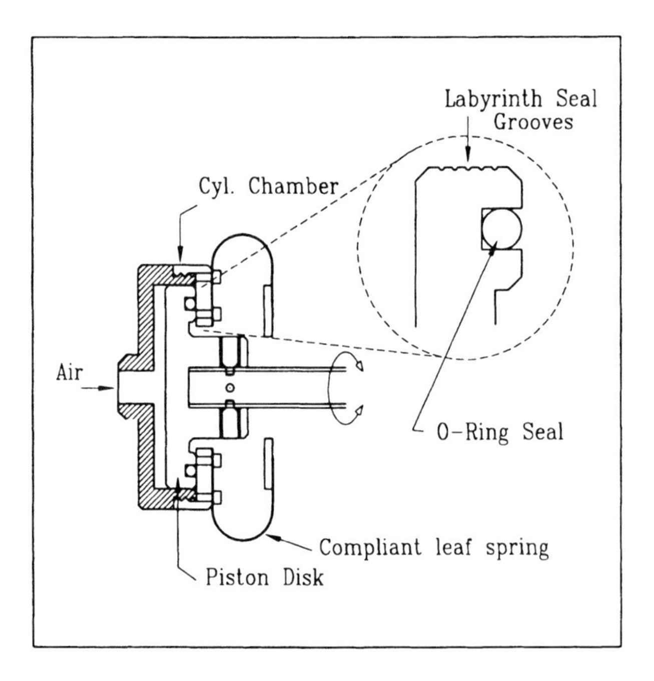

Figure 2.10. The locking mechanism of wrists joints.

however due to possible leakage, are not suitable for surgical environment. The pneumatic locks are considered the solution which satisfies all the requirements. However they are relatively larger than hydraulic locks due to lower operating pressure (i.e. maximum of 7 Bar$\approx 0.7MPa$).

The internal design of locks for the wrists joints, and the arms are shown in Fig. 2.10 and Fig. 2.11 respectively. The designs consist of a piston disk and cylinder chamber, which each are connected to one of the two links of the joint. When the cylinder chamber is pressurized, the piston disk is frictionally engaged with the bottom of the chamber. The frictional locking torque in both cases can be approximated by :

$$\tau_{fric} = \mu . F_{Cyl} . D/2 = \mu . (P_{air} . A_{cyl}) . D/2 = \mu . P_{air} . \pi D^3/8$$

Where, D is the diameter of cylinder, P_{air} is the operating air pressure, and μ is the Coulomb coefficient of friction (minimum value assumed to be ≈ 0.2 for unlubricated metal to metal contact). By applying the above values of μ, τ and P, the diameters of cylinders for the wrists and arms locks can be calculated as 53 and 80mm respectively, which is relatively compact for the design.

When the cylinder chamber is pressurized, the cylinder and the piston would have a small axial movement (i.e. 0.2-0.5mm) with respect to each other in order to get frictionally engaged. The freedom of movement for

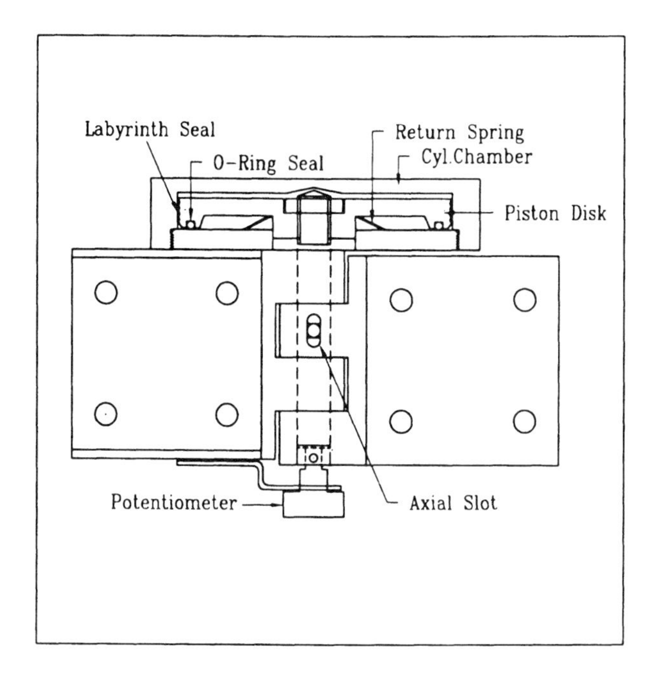

Figure 2.11. The locking mechanism of arms joints.

the relative axial movement is assured by: a) the compliance of the spring links in the wrists locks (which holds the chamber rigidly in all directions except the axial direction, so the chamber can move slightly in the axial direction, Fig. 2.10), and b) the axial slots in the arms locks (so the piston disk and its shaft can move slightly Fig. 2.11).

In order to minimize the frictional torque due to seals (e.g. O-ring or lip seal on the periphery of the piston), the sealing is provided by : a) a *labyrinth* seal consisting of several parallel grooves on the side of the piston (which causes gradual pressure drop through each groove), and b) the *O-ring* seal at the bottom surface of disk which prevents any final leak.

5. PROTOTYPE DEVELOPMENT AND EVALUATION

Based on the synthesis of the wrist and arm mechanisms, a prototype of the laparoscopic stand has been developed (Fig. 2.12). The arms are supported by a single vertical column which also provides the vertical adjustment of the arms through a lead screw and handle mechanism.

The stand performs all the initial design requirements of a) having spherical movement at the remote center of rotation, b) reaching the entire work-space (i.e.$350 \times 500 mm^2$ for the two arms), c) locking effec-

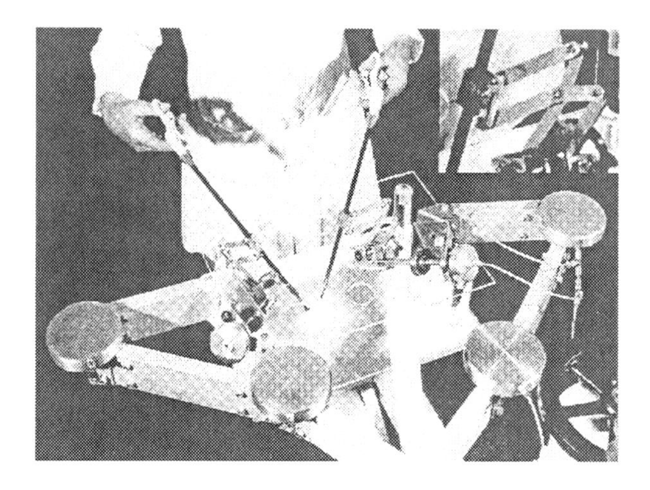

Figure 2.12. The laparoscopic stand with two arms.

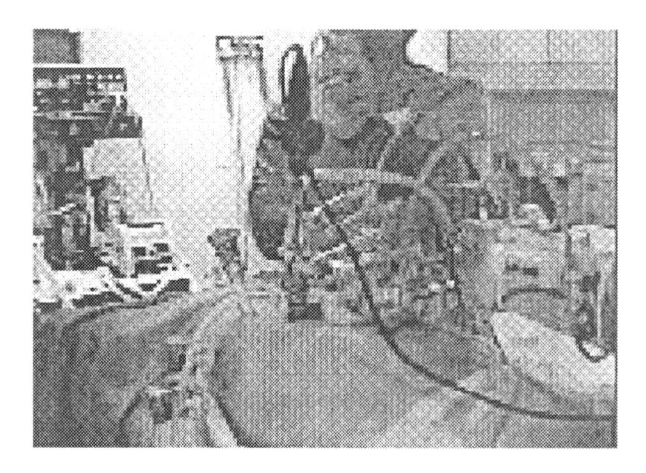

Figure 2.13. Experimenting with the laparoscopic stand in Jack Bell Centre.

tively all the joints (both kinds of joints for the wrists and arms) with sufficient stiffness, d) being able to manipulate and move freely the arms and wrists for their entire prescribed range of movements.

The prototype has been evaluated at the animal surgical laboratory of Jack Bell Centre[62] during laparoscopic training sessions of surgeons. Some of the positive comments are:

- The ability to move and lock the laparoscopic tools/instruments freely over the incision points during the operation compared to the conventional positioners[2] (which can only hold stationary tools).

- The size of wrist mechanisms did not create interference problem with other tools, or with each other over the body.
- The locking of joints were sufficient under the loads (e.g. weight of laparoscope or stiffness of the abdominal wall), and firm without any excessive backlash/play.
- The range of angular movements of the wrists was large enough to accommodate for all surgical movements.

On the other hand, the negative aspects are:

- The mounting base of the stand (comprising of a frame attached on the top of a pallet-jack for mobility) was not compatible with the base of surgical bed, causing positioning and reaching problems for the arms over the incision points.
- The column structure and its base takes too much space on the bed-side, and is not acceptable for the surgical environment.
- The tool holders at the tip of wrist mechanisms should be in the form of a grasper, so that the tools attachment to the wrist can be performed fast with relative ease.
- The whole design and especially positioning arms require further miniaturization in order to become compatible with space requirements of the surgical work-space.

6. DISCUSSIONS

The prototype was designed and developed for evaluation of the design concepts related to the wrist and arm mechanisms. Although it functioned successfully, and met the initial design objectives, it requires further developmental enhancements. By studying the experimental feedbacks, the following possible changes and improvements can be summarized :

- The reachable space for both arms (i.e.$500 \times 350mm$) was initially chosen rather conservatively to cover the whole chest and abdominal area. However, as a result of the experimentation it is essential to miniaturize the prototype further. Consequently the actual minimum size of the reachable space for different procedures should be determined and to be used as the initial design parameters. Any reduction in this area would result in direct proportional reduction in the overall size of the arms. This can provide $30 - 40\%$ reduction in the size of each arm.

- In the case of miniaturization of wrist mechanisms, the parameter L_1 can be substantially reduced if the current trocar design is modified with less overall length. This can be implemented, resulting up to 40% in reduction of sizes for the wrist mechanisms.

- Another general method to reduce the size of joints, and linkages cross sections, is by choosing higher strength material. For example, instead of aluminum in the prototype stainless steel can be a good substitute for this purpose.

- The overall diameter of locks at each joint can be reduced if the above size reductions are applied.

- One of the main concerns of surgeons regarding the stand was its space requirement along the bed-side, which can be addressed by revising the design in either of the following ways:

    1. To use an over head positioning arm such as Type 12 (Fig. 2.5) as described in Sec.2.2.

    2. To compromise the naturally balanced SCARA arms with some other unbalanced arm types, such as 82 or 83 (Fig. 2.5), in order to be able to mount each individual arm to the bed-side. This modular design of each arm as a separate unit without any need to a separate mounting base is further described in the final chapter as part of future work.

Chapter 3

FLEXIBLE STEM GRASPERS

Since the earliest times, humans have used tools to extend their ability to reach and move objects. One main application of tools has been to move objects for the purpose of a) *positioning* with three degrees of freedom (DOF), and b)*orienting* with an additional three DOF. The six DOF of the movement is defined as *manipulation* of the object [92].

In some tasks, due to the *remoteness* of the site, the object manipulations can not be performed directly. The remoteness could be due to: 1) *a physical barrier* (e.g. protective walls of a nuclear facility, or a high temperature furnace), or 2) *the distance* (e.g. in the case of deep under-water, or space exploration).

Based on the interpretation of the definition, laparoscopy could also be considered as a *remote* operation, which must be performed behind the *barrier* of abdominal wall. Moreover, the port of entry at the abdominal wall acts as a spherical pivot which permits 4 DOF (3 rotational around the three mutually perpendicular axes XYZ, and one translational along the Z axis, Fig. 3.1), for surgical *extenders*. The term *extender* is defined as any surgical instrument being used to extend/transfer the capabilities of the surgeon (such as, manipulating/cutting the tissue) to the surgical site, or transfer sensations (e.g. force/tactile signals) from the surgical site to the surgeon.

One aspect of the dexterity problem associated with laparoscopic surgery arises from the fact that the present rigid stem extenders can only approach the surgical site with some fixed orientation (determined by the connecting line between the position of the surgical site and the port of entry). Lack of 2 DOF does not allow the desired orientation of the surgical tool and prevents the surgeon from having the required dexterity and agility at the surgical site. By adding rotary joints on the

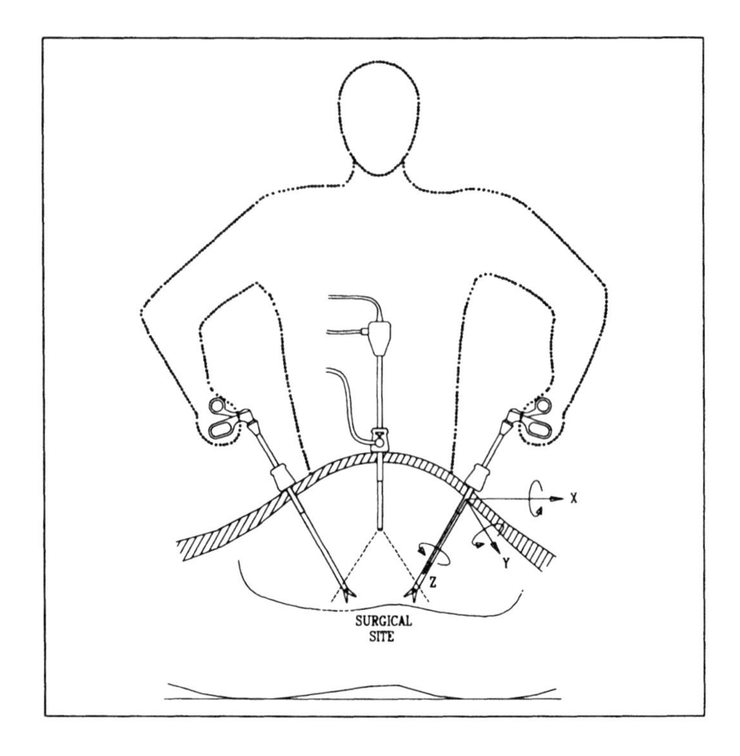

Figure 3.1. Body posture of the surgeon with rigid stem graspers.

stem, the required *internal* DOF in orienting the tool can be achieved, hence providing more dexterity for the surgeon.

On the other hand, the dexterity of the surgeon is also affected by another *external* aspect related to the awkward and un-relaxed body posture of the surgeon. This is due to the fixed outward orientation of rigid stem tools from the surgical site through the ports of entry on the abdomen. This fixed orientation of tools usually puts the surgeon in an awkward body posture (Fig. 3.1) for the duration of the operation, which could affect his/her precision and dexterity greatly. However, if the stem has additional rotary joints inside the abdomen (as internal DOF), then the location of ports of entry could be selected independent of the tools orientation, so that the surgeon's body posture is closer to a normal/relaxed state (Fig. 3.2). In other words, we want to decouple the *internal* requirement (i.e. the desired orientation of extender's tip) from the *external* requirement (i.e. the normal body posture), by creating additional DOF on the stem.

There have been a lot of developments in the field of the design and development of endoscopic flexible stems in the last few years [58] [59] [71] [81] [95]. Also, there are commercially available graspers such as,

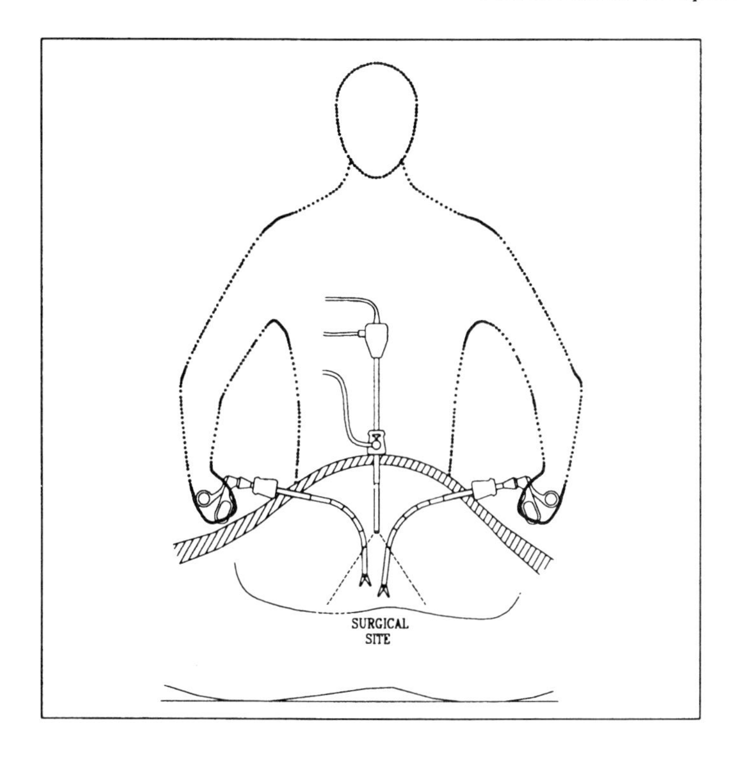

Figure 3.2. Body posture of the surgeon with flexible stem graspers.

"Steerable Fiberscopes" by Karl Storz-Endoskope[80], or endoscopic retractors and graspers as "EndoFlex" instruments series by Surgical Innovation Ltd.[84], as well as industrial patents [44] [56] [57] for flexible endoscopes.

Although the above provides detailed information about different design possibilities, they are all dealing with *special* designs with specific design focus, and there is a lack of *general* study of flexible laparoscopic extenders with wider design approach. The objectives of the design can be stated as:

- Development of a general type synthesis of joints rather than focusing on one type.
- Formulation of the workspace requirements for laparoscopic extenders inside the abdominal cavity.
- Comparative study of different designs in search of the optimal design (s).

In order to address the above issues, the attempt in this chapter is to develop a systematic approach for the design of joints and their actuation mechanism (Sec. 1). Also, we define and formulate the dexterous workspace for laparoscopic extenders with a flexible stem for finding the optimum design (Sec. 2, and 3). Finally, integration aspects of the designs and their evaluation are discussed in sections 4, and 5 .

1. SYNTHESIS OF FLEXIBLE LAPAROSCOPIC EXTENDERS

For the type synthesis of the flexible stem, first we need to know what type of joint provides the *range* of rotary motion, and the required DOF. In general, there are two classes of rotary joints a) revolute joints (with 1 DOF), and b) spherical joints (with up to 3 DOF). The challenge and difficulty lies in the design of these joints on a stem which a) has a diameter of only 5-10 mm, b) has to be actuated deep inside the body, and c) the mechanical design still should provide some room for the linkages and connectors to pass through the joint(s) and to the other moving elements[1] or receptors[2] at the other end of the extender.

However, there could be many variations in designs. Here three new designs are studied, where two are revolute, and one is spherical types.

Type.1- Single-revolute joint design : This design is based on a 4-bar linkage mechanism, that actuates a single revolute joint on the stem (Fig. 3.3, for more details see Ap.B, Fig.B1). This can provide a simple and robust joint mechanism with one additional DOF. The difficulty is in the designing of a single revolute joint that can provide all the wide range of rotation (e.g. from 0° to 120°). This design constraint could be the major cause that none of the research groups have worked on this type, and only one commercial product (i.e. a tissue stapler by Ethicon) has used this design with very limited joint rotation (0° to 45°). However, in our new design (Fig. 3.3), by moving the axis of the main joint to one extreme side of the stem, as well as by using concentric tubes for the actuation of the 4-bar linkage mechanism , both problems of actuation and accessibility to the end of the tool are resolved, while providing the joint with a wide angular deflection up to 120°. The combination of this design and the rotating grasper head (with one additional DOF, described in Sec.4, Fig. 3.13), provides a viable design with a total of 6 DOF (Fig. 3.15).

Type.2- Multi-revolute joints design : This is the most applied type of design among different research groups [64][71], as well as

[1] e.g. grasper, or stapler, etc.

[2] e.g. fiber optics bundles for the objective lens of the laparoscope.

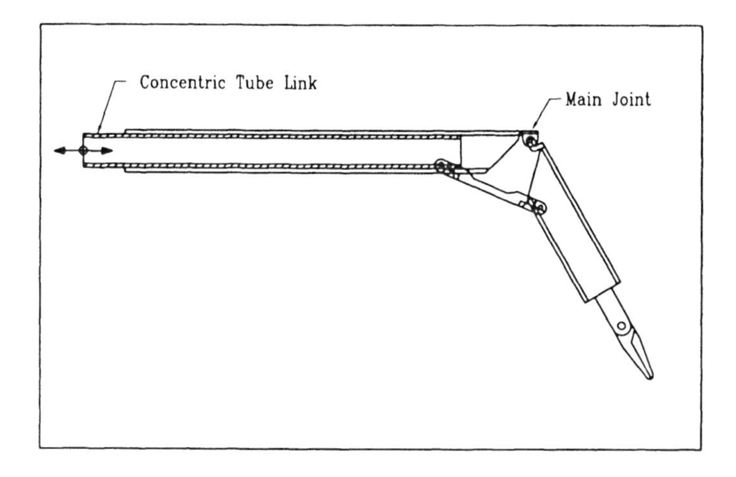

Figure 3.3. 4-bar linkage actuated single joint design

commercial developers [56][84]. This is due to the fact that the angular deflection of each joint is quite limited (30° to 45°), so to provide sufficient articulation of the extender at its tip, there must be several joints in series (minimum of 2 to 4 joints). This creates another challenge for actuating all the joints simultaneously. Among the above developers almost all are using some form of tendon actuation mechanism. However, in the proposed design of this chapter, another more unconventional approach for actuation is employed. It consists of left/right handed lead screws that drives two nuts connected to each link (Fig. 3.4, for more details see Ap.B, Fig.B2). To transfer the actuation motion to all the joints, the end of each successive shaft are connected in series by helical spring couplings. The input rotation of the first lead screw actuates all the connecting joints to the maximum angle of 45°. Another additional DOF of the rotary grasping head (described in Sec. 4), provides a total of 6 DOF for the integrated design (Fig. 3.16).

Type.3- Multi-spherical joints design :

A spherical joint can provide up to 3 DOF, which makes it attractive for application in laparoscopic extenders. However, problems such as the actuation, locking, and controlled motion of such spherical joint, have prevented the use of this type of joint for laparoscopic extenders. In this work, the possibility of the design of multi-spherical joints actuated by tendon wires is investigated as an alternative design for laparoscopic extenders (Fig. 3.5, for more details see Ap.B, Fig.B3). However, there are some design challenges which can be stated as:

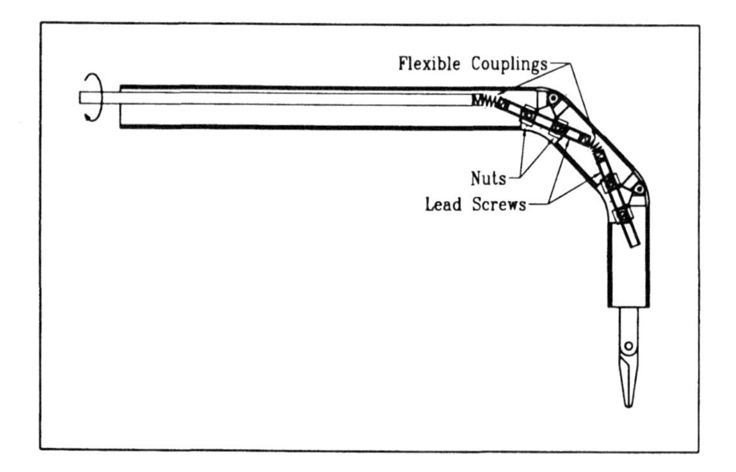

Figure 3.4. Lead screw actuated multi-revolute joints design

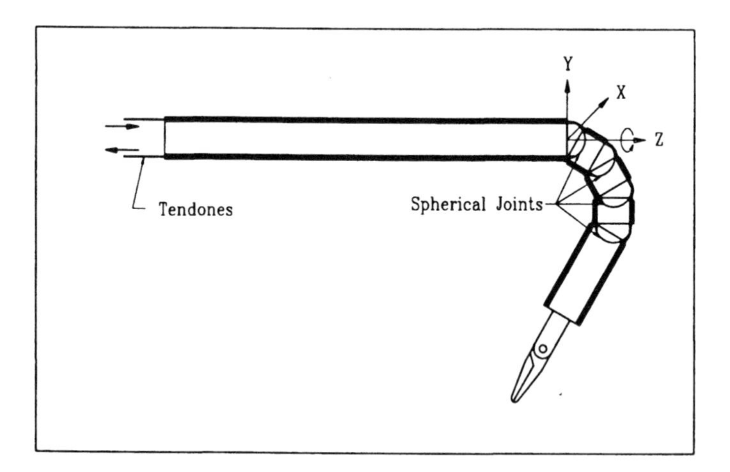

Figure 3.5. Tendon actuated multi-spherical joints design

- To access the end of the tool, there should exist a central bore that, when the joint is actuated, will be partially blocked as the spherical joints rotate with respect to each other. In order to have a minimum central passage (e.g.3-5mm in the case of our prototype with O.D.18mm), the joints' deflection must be limited to the range of 20° to 30°. As a result, at least 3 to 5 joints are required in order to provide sufficient dexterity at the tip of the extender.

- Each spherical joint in this design has only 2 DOF since the tendons prevent rotation around Z axis (Fig. 3.5), which is actuated by two sets of double tendons near the periphery of the stem. On the other hand, the high number of joints creates redundancy in the actuation. For example by actuating the tendons there will be control over the orientation of the end point, but there will not be control over the orientation of each individual intermediate joints. The problem can be addressed partially by installing spring wires parallel to tendons which are attached to the base of the stem. This causes the joints to be almost synchronized and deflect uniformly as well as returning to an initial straight state after the tendons' tension are released. In addition, by adding a rotary grasping head (similar to Fig. 3.13), the maximum DOF of such an extender inside the abdominal cavity would be 3 DOF (plus the other 4 DOF at the port of entry, the total would be 7 DOF).

- The rotation of spherical joints is caused by differential tension in the tendons, and their locking can be obtained by equal high tension in all tendons (causing locking due to Coulomb friction at the joints). In this regard, friction models of spherical socket-ball joints (as well as revolute pin joints) [30]for controlled actuation and locking purposes should be developed (see Ap.A). However, the work here is limited only to the control of the movement of tendons through a mechanical type joy-stick (Fig. 3.17) for manual control.

For further comparative study of above designs, the reachable and dexterous workspace for laparoscopy is formulated in the following section.

2. LAPAROSCOPIC WORKSPACE FORMULATION

For any manipulator or robotic arm, being able to reach a "prescribed workspace", is an important and essential requirement. This also has to be done early in the design stage. Here we defined the *Dexterous Workspace* as a subset of *Reachable Workspace* where the grasping head can reach with any arbitrary orientation[65]. This classification is very useful and relevant to the design of the flexible stem graspers. In this section, first we define the *Reachable*, and *Dexterous Workspaces* in laparoscopic surgery. Then a general parametric model of flexible extenders is formulated. A new dexterity measure of the single and multi-joint designs is then examined.

As was mentioned, in laparoscopy due to kinematic constraints at the incision point, not only the movement of the tool is limited to 4DOF, but also its range of motion. For instance, in the case of rotational

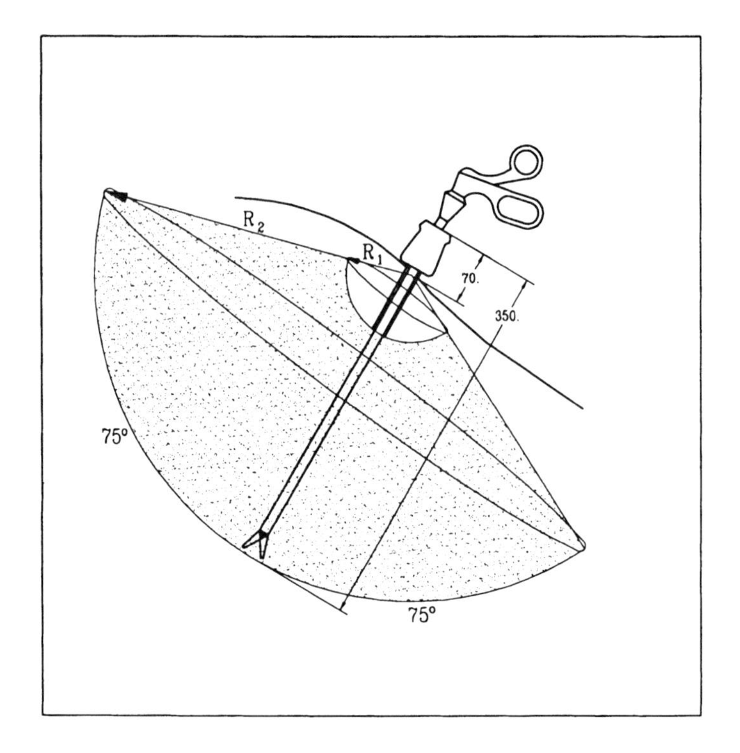

Figure 3.6. Laparoscopic reachable workspace

movement around X and Y axis (Fig. 3.1), due to limited compliance of the abdominal wall, it is possible to rotate the tool only in the range of $\pm 75°$ around these axes (Fig. 3.6). Also, the maximum penetration of laparoscopic tool is limited to its total length minus the external length of trocar (i.e. $R_2 = 350mm - 70mm = 280mm$, Fig. 3.6). Finally, the internal extension of trocar creates additional limit to the minimum penetrating length of laparoscopic tool (i.e. $R_1 = 80mm$, Fig. 3.6). This makes the *laparoscopic reachable workspace* to be a conical section bounded by two spheres with radiuses $R_1 = 80mm$, and $R_2 = 280mm$, with the total cone angle of 150° (Fig. 3.6).

On the other hand, the flexible extender can be considered generally as a long stem of length L with N joints where intermediate linkages have the size of L_N, and the end link with grasper has the size of L_E (Fig. 3.7). In general, in the plane of extender, to reach a point in the reachable workspace, with the depth coordinates of $[R, \Theta]$, and orientation φ, the stem has to deflect to an angle α , and penetrate length L (as shown in Fig. 3.7) beyond the last joint, while the multi-joints are deflected each by the equal angle β.

The variables used in this formulation can be defined as:

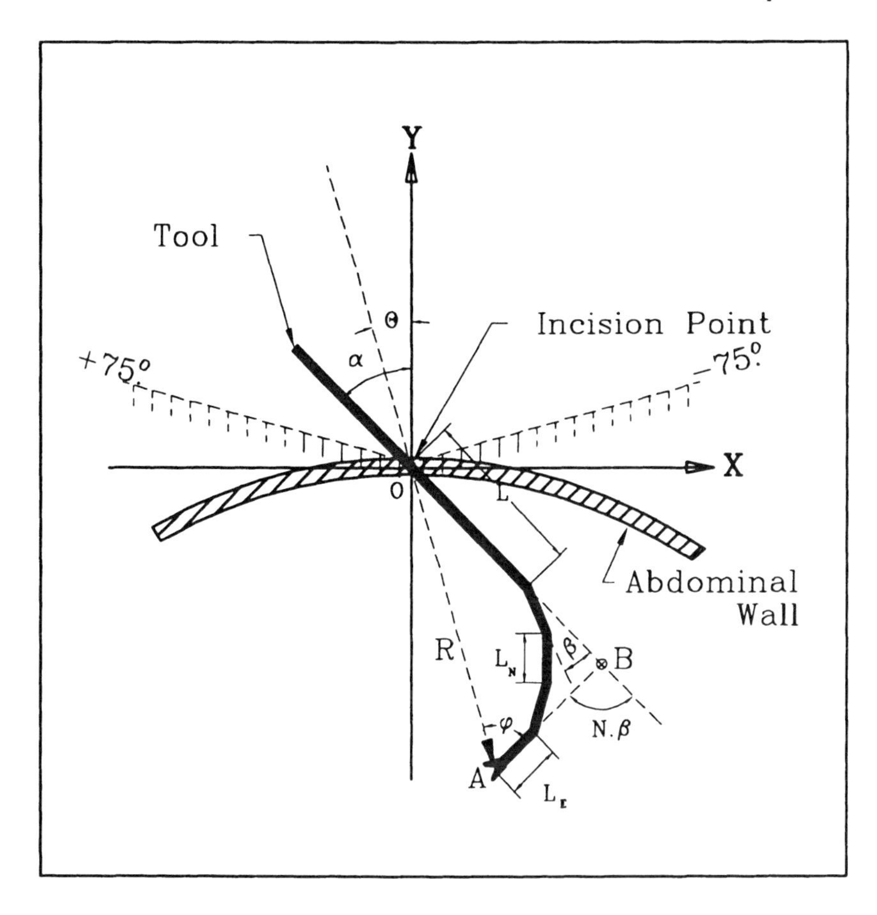

Figure 3.7. Endoscopic workspace of a flexible stem tool.

a) Workspace Variables: R, Θ, φ

b) Design Variables: L_N, L_E, β, N.

The constraints on the design and the objective function can be defined as :

I) Inequality Constraints:

Reachable Workspace :	$80 \leq R \leq 280$;	penetration range of surgical extender.
	$\alpha \leq 75°$;	flexibility range of abdominal wall.
Design Parameters :	$L_E \geq l_e$;	minimum size of intermediate links.
	$L_N \geq l_n$;	minimum size of end link.
	$\beta \leq \beta_{max}$;	maximum range of joints deflection.
	$N \leq n$;	feasible range of joints number.

Based on the three types of designs which are previously discussed, the parameters β_{max}, l_n, l_e, and n are the limiting values of variables β, L_N, L_E, and N, that are defined in Table 3.1 :

Table 3.1. The design variables of 3 types of flexible stem.

Type	β_{max}	l_n	l_e	n
1	90.	0.	70.	1
2	45.	28.	60.	2-4
3	30.	10.	50.	3-5

II) Equality Constraints:

For a flexible stem to reach point A in the reachable workspace, with coordinates $[R, \Theta]$, and orientation φ, the kinematic model of the flexible extender as a multi-linkage system results in the following geometric equality constraints:

$$L \sin \alpha + L_N[\sin(\alpha - \beta) + ... + \sin(\alpha - (N-1)\beta)] + L_E \sin(\alpha - N\beta) = R \sin \Theta$$

and

$$L \cos \alpha + L_N[\cos(\alpha - \beta) + ... + \cos(\alpha - (N-1)\beta)] + L_E \cos(\alpha - N\beta) = R \cos \Theta$$

Or in the following form :

$$\begin{bmatrix} L \\ L_N \\ L_E \end{bmatrix}^T \begin{bmatrix} \sin \alpha & \cos \alpha \\ \sum_{i=1}^{N-1} \sin(\alpha - i\beta) & \sum_{i=1}^{N-1} \cos(\alpha - i\beta) \\ \sin(\alpha - N\beta) & \cos(\alpha - N\beta) \end{bmatrix} = R \begin{bmatrix} \sin \Theta \\ \cos \Theta \end{bmatrix}^T$$

III) Objective Function:

In the planar formulation of the laparoscopic workspace (Fig. 3.7), we defined three workspace variables (or coordinates)$[R, \Theta, \varphi]$. The objective is to find the maximum approach angle φ for any given point in the reachable space$[R, \Theta]$. This is casted as an optimization problem where the objective function is to maximize φ, for different values of R, and Θ. The objective function can be formulated by geometry of the triangle OAB (Fig. 3.7), where the angle $N.\beta = \varphi + \alpha - \Theta$, which can be rearranged as:

$$\textbf{Maximize: } \varphi = N.\beta + \Theta - \alpha$$

Which is solved numerically in the next section for all the points covering the entire reachable workspace with a small spatial increments as defined in the section.

3. OPTIMAL DESIGN OF THE FLEXIBLE STEM

The proposed formulation has been solved for 546 points in the reachable workspace (i.e. a 26×21 mesh of $3°$ increments in Θ direction, and

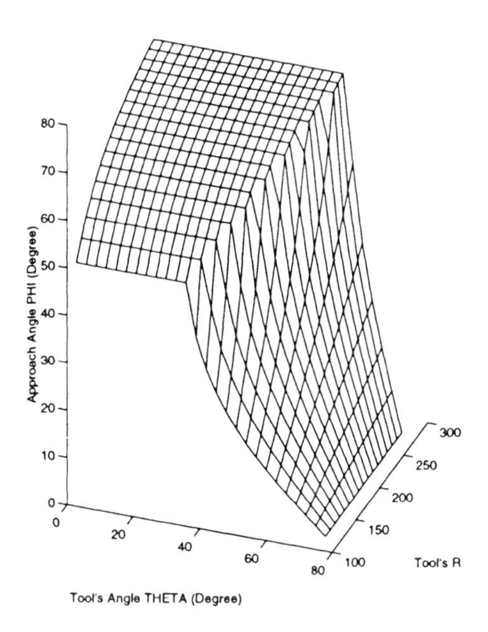

Figure 3.8. The workspace of Type 1.

$10mm$ in R direction). In the case of Type 1, the results are plotted for φ vs. Θ, and R as shown in Fig. 3.8. In this figure it can be seen that, φ increases as R increases (this is expected since the tool would have more room for bending as it penetrates deeper). However, as Θ increases, φ remains constant first, and then it decreases sharply as soon as the base of the stem reaches the angular limit of α (i.e. $75°$). Same trend for φ is observed for all of the designs, with different ranges and maximum limits of φ. In some cases, the range of φ is from 0 to a maximum value of $120°$.

In general, a manipulator is defined to be *dexterous* at a specific point in its reachable workspace, if it can reach the point from any orientation. This definition of *dexterity* can be modified for applications that do not require all the possible set of orientations at a specific point in the reachable workspace. For example, when the end-effector of a manipulator is approaching a point on a solid surface, its orientation relative to the normal vector of the surface can vary in the range of zero up to $\pm 90°$ theoretically. Practically, the maximum deviation from the normal vector is even less than $90°$ in this case, due to the interference of the joints and the side of the end-effector with the surface. This is similar to the case we have in laparoscopy, when the flexible extender approaches the surgical site. The maximum dexterity the extender can have is in

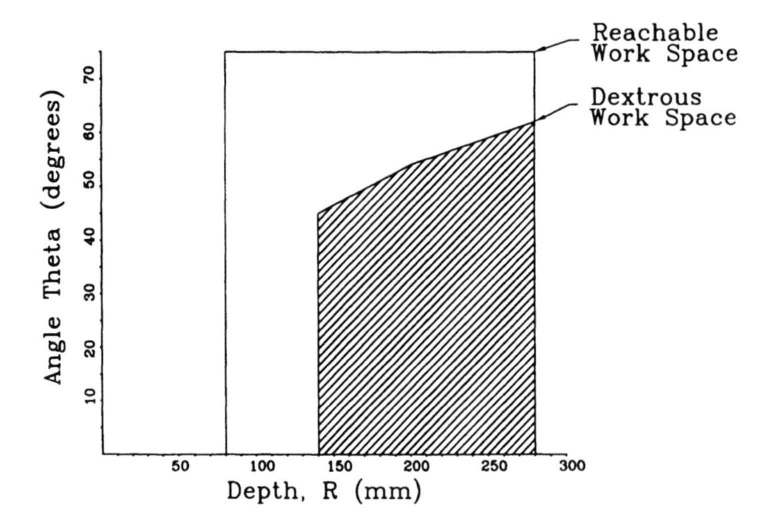

Figure 3.9. Type 1 with 1 joint.

the range of 0 to 90°. However, a flexible extender could be considered *dexterous* if it can approach a given coordinate$[R, \Theta]$ with a minimum approach angle φ_{min} in the range of 30° – 90°[3]. As an example, an average value of $\varphi_{min} = 60°$ is chosen to be the minimum requirement for the approach angle. Therefore by choosing the minimum limit of 60° for angle φ, in Fig. 3.8, only the portion of workspace which is above the limit (i.e. $\varphi \geq 60°$) can be considered as the *dexterous workspace.* The projected view of this dexterous workspace (i.e. R vs. Θ) is shown in Fig. 3.9 in comparison to the total reachable workspace.

The same procedure is performed for design Type 2 with 2,3, and 4 joints, and for Type 3 with 3,4, and 5 joints, as shown in Fig. 3.10, and 3.11 respectively. This provides the basis for comparison of their dexterous workspace, with the number of joints as the criterion for the type synthesis of these different types of designs.

In order to compare the performance of multi-linkage systems locally (i.e. at some specific location) or globally (i.e. in the entire reachable workspace), performance measures are used in the literature to quantify different performance characteristics of the system. For example, Yoshikawa[98], introduced $m = |det(J)|$ (where J is the Jacobian of the manipulator) as a measure of manipulability for comparing manipulating forces, or Doel and Pai[20], have defined several new measures for inertia, and redundancy of multi-linkage systems.

[3]Depending on the required level of dexterity this limit could vary in that range (i.e. 30° – 90°).

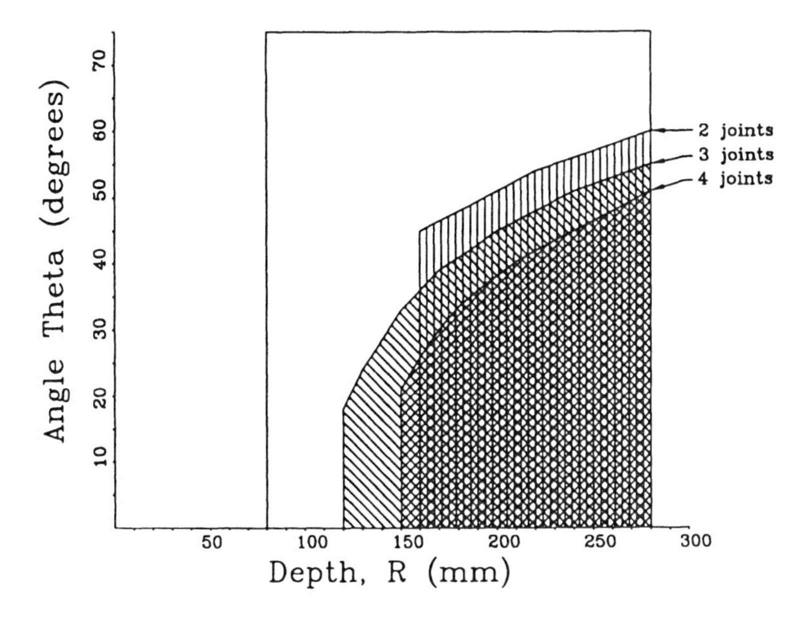

Figure 3.10. Type 2 with 2, 3, 4 joints.

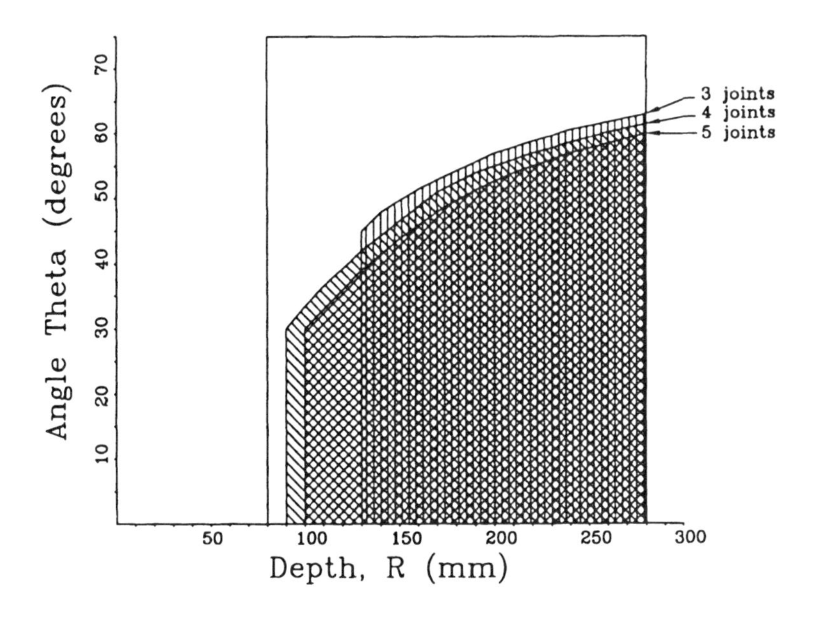

Figure 3.11. Type 3 with 3, 4, 5 joints.

To be able to compare dexterous workspaces of designs with different number of joints, and to evaluate different types of designs with respect to each other, a new *Dexterity Measure* is defined. This measure is

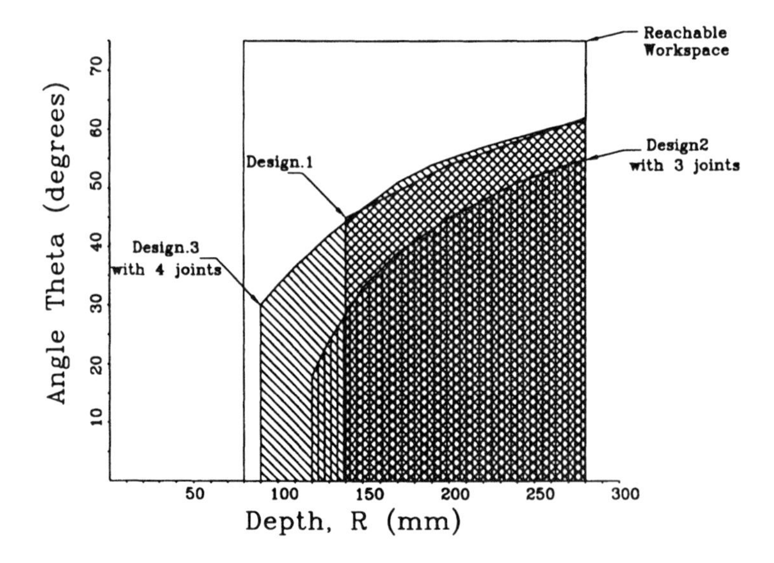

Figure 3.12. Dexterous workspace of Types 1, 2, and 3.

the ratio between areas of dexterous and reachable workspaces occupy (Fig. 3.9):

$$\text{Dexterity Measure} = \frac{\text{Dexterous Workspace Area}}{\text{Reachable Workspace Area}} \tag{3.1}$$

For example, the ratio of the shaded area to the rectangular area is the dexterity measure of Type 1 (the planar workspace shown in Fig. 3.9). The ratio is dimensionless and always between 0 and 1, since the dexterous workspace is always a subset of reachable space. This provides a global dexterity measure that indicates what percentage of the reachable workspace is dexterous. Furthermore, since the reachable workspace is the same for all three types (Fig. 3.12), the ratio could be used for comparison of their dexterity with respect to each other, as shown in Table 3.2 .

Table 3.2. Dexterity measures of Types 1, 2, and 3.

Type	1	2			3		
Joints, N	1	2	3	4	3	4	5
Dexterity Measure	**51%**	43%	**45%**	34%	56%	**64%**	59%

The formulation of dexterity measure could have also been based on the ratio of the actual volume of dexterous workspace, divided by the volume of reachable workspace. In this case the volume of a workspace (Fig. 3.6) would be :

$$V = \int_{R_1}^{R_2} \int_0^{\theta} 2\pi R \sin\theta R d\theta dR$$

Taking the simple case of a plain conical workspace where θ is a constant and independent of R, the above integral reduces to :

$$V = \frac{2\pi}{3}(R_2^3 - R_1^3)(1 - \cos\theta)$$

From the above equation, it is evident that the workspace volume is a function of R to the third power. This makes the volume-based dexterity measure very biased toward tools that have better dexterity at greater depths although they do not have any dexterity at shallow depths (e.g. design 2 with 2 joints for $R \leq 160mm$, or design 3 with 3 joints for $R \leq 130mm$, Fig. 3.10, and Fig. 3.11 respectively). On the other hand, the dexterity measure used in this section based on "workspace area" (Eq. 3.1) is equally related to the first power of both R, and θ, hence providing a non-biased measure with respect to the workspace variables.

Based on the calculated dexterity measures of Table 3.2, the following conclusions regarding different types and their number synthesis could be reached :

- The optimum number of joints, to provide the highest dexterity, for design Type 2, is 3 joints.

- The optimum number of joints, to provide the highest dexterity, for design Type 3, is 4 joints.

- Type 3 is the most dexterous compared to the other two designs.

- With the exception of relatively shallow depths of operation (where $R < 130mm$), Type 1 provides almost the same dexterity measure as Type 3 (Fig. 3.12), while in comparison, it is much simpler in design, and easier to actuate.

- Type 2 does not have any dexterity advantage compared to the other two designs.

In the following section, other mechanical design features related to the grasping head of laparoscopic flexible extenders are discussed.

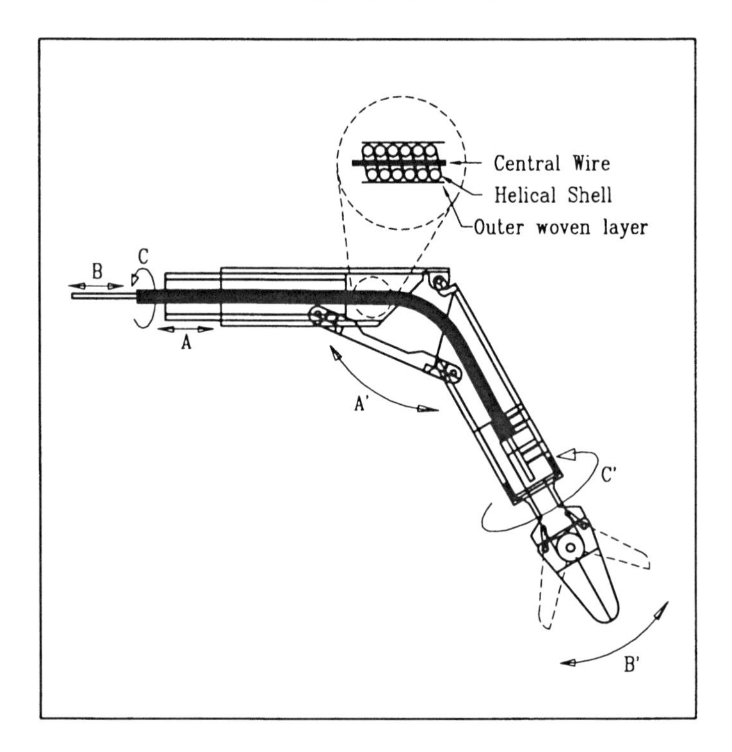

Figure 3.13. Functional movements of grasping head by flexible shaft design.

4. FEATURES OF THE MECHANICAL DESIGN

For any laparoscopic extender with a flexible stem, in order to be able to function effectively (beside the flexing motion of the joints on the stem), it is essential that its grasping head would be able to have the required movements/actuations. There are two functional movements which are required for the grasping head as follows :

1. The actuation of the grasper: Usually this is a reciprocating scissors-like motion of a set of jaws for grasping, cutting, dissecting, etc.

2. The axial rotation of the head: For the proper alignment of the jaws of the grasper with the tissue or the needle, the grasping head requires rotary motion around Z-axis (Fig. 3.1). In current laparoscopic graspers, this function is performed by the rotation of the rigid stem itself. However, in the case of flexible stem extenders, the axial rotation of the grasping head can not be performed from the

base of stem[4]. Hence, the rotation of the tool-head can only be performed locally by having one additional axial rotary joint (i.e. axis C', Fig. 3.13) after the flexing joint (s) on the stem (e.g. joint A'). This provides one additional DOF for orientation of the extender.

A design challenge is to transfer the above two functional movements (i.e. grasping, and the head rotation), from the handle to the grasping head considering the spatial limitation at the flexing joint (s). There could also be numerous design variations for this motion transmission (e.g. by wire, or hydraulic lines, etc.). A compact and suitable solution that can transfer both movements on a single cable (2-3 mm in diameter) is a push-pull flexible shaft design (Fig. 3.13). Basically the flexible shaft consists of a central flexible element (i.e. usually a spring wire), which provides the linear reciprocating motion (for the grasping action), and a helical outer shell (like a helical extension spring) that can transfer the rotary motion to the head[74].

The additional advantage of this flexible shaft design is that the transmission of the motion and the force between the handle and the grasping head is achieved without exerting any significant load on the flexing joint (s) on the stem. This design has been successfully developed on a prototype with the single-revolute joint design as shown in Fig. 3.13 (for more details see Ap.B, Fig.B4), which can also be applied to the multi-spherical joints design (Type.3, Fig. 3.5, and 3.17). However, in the case of multi-revolute joints design (Type.2, Fig. 3.4, and 3.16), the passages through the joints are not wide enough to allow the flexible shaft to pass through. Hence, for the development of Type 2 (Fig. 3.4), another design consisting of a tension wire is used to close a normally-open spring-loaded grasper, as well as to rotate the grasping head (Fig. 3.14). This design, although very compact, suffers from the following limitations:

- Excessive friction in the grasping movement due to the contact, as well as its bending at each joint.
- Low stiffness and excessive backlash in the rotational movement of the head.
- Exerting external load on the flexing joints of the stem, due to bends in the tension wire, which causes undesired jerking motion of the grasping head (due to inherent clearance at each pivoting joint).

[4]since the orientation of the tool-head is different from the tool-stem due to the actuation of flexing joints.

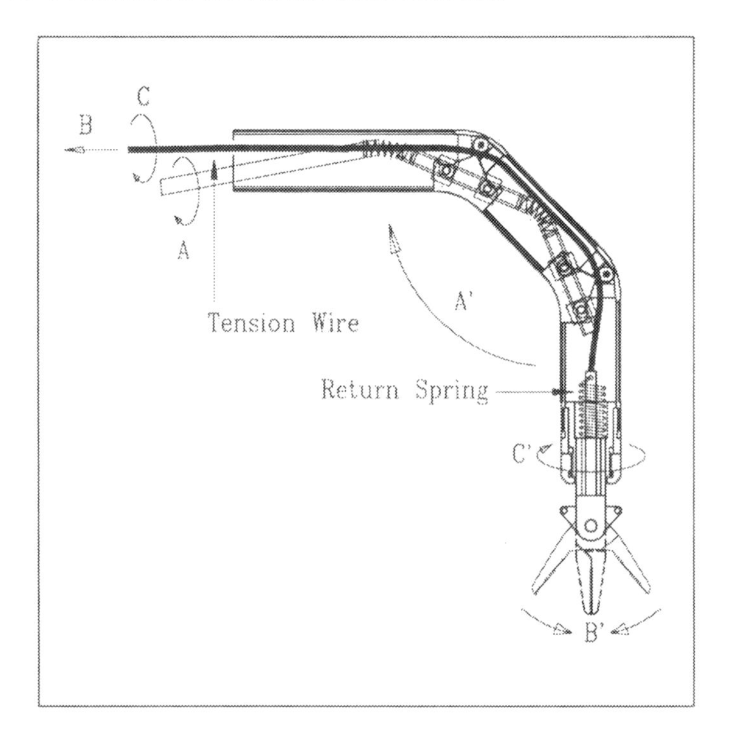

Figure 3.14. Functional movements of grasping head by tensional wire design.

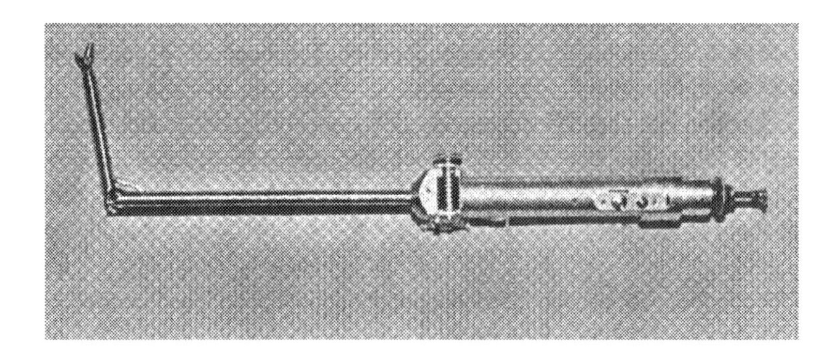

Figure 3.15. Prototype of Type 1 design with 6 DOF.

5. DISCUSSION

- **Type 1** satisfies all the functional requirements of a) having a flexible stem with sufficient dexterity (in this case it has 120° articulation at the joint), b) having the additional DOF for the tip of the tool to rotate around its central axis while the joint at the stem is articulated, c) actuating the grasper through the articulated joint, and d) having a maximum diameter of only 10mm. However, for clinical trial, further

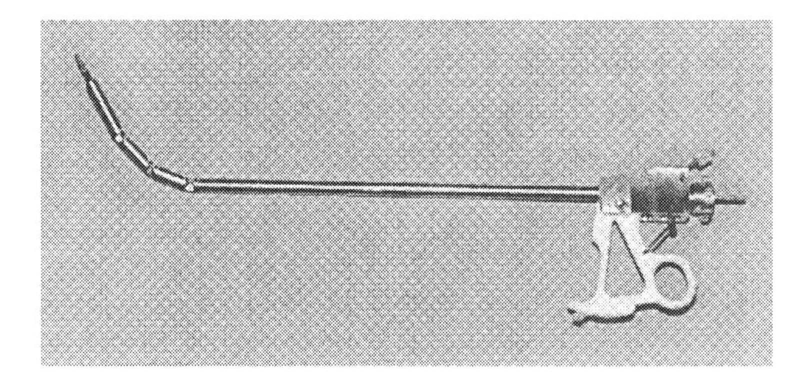

Figure 3.16. Prototype of Type 2 design with 6 DOF.

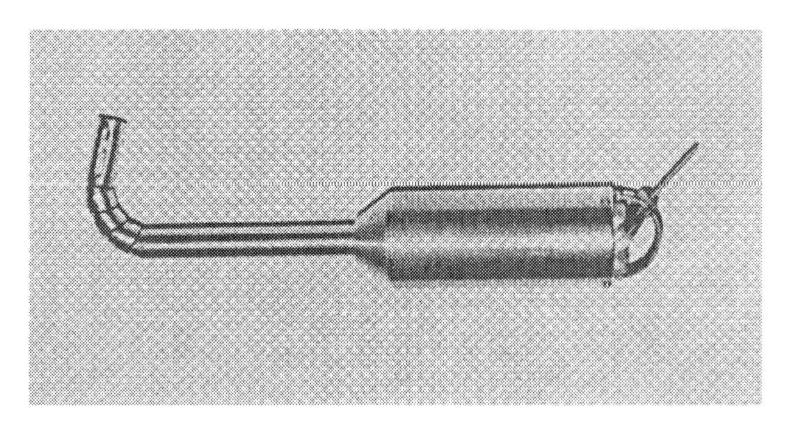

Figure 3.17. Experimental prototype of Type 3 design with 7 possible DOF.

developmental work is required to enhance the current prototype by reducing the length of the end-link (i.e. L_e) from 50mm to 20-30mm, (Fig. 3.7, Fig. 3.15). The new prototype would be compatible with the limited space inside the abdominal cavity, and would be able to rotate its stem to reach the entire dexterous workspace (Fig. 3.9).

Size L_e could not be reduced in the current prototype due to a) the relatively large diameter of the available flexible shaft (i.e. 3.5mm), which requires a larger bending radius, and subsequently longer end-link (i.e. L_e). However, by using more compact flexible shafts available from a recent supplier[74] it is possible to overcome both of the above-mentioned problems.

- **Type 2** is not as dexterous compared to other two types due to larger size of its linkages. Also, it is not robust, and requires frequent repair and maintenance because of its high number of moving parts.

Although the actuation of its joints was possible, but very much prone to fatigue, as well as clogging at the lead screws. Therefore this design was abandoned, and is not considered for further development.

- **Type 3** proved to be a viable design with high DOF and dexterity. However, it has to be further miniaturized in order to be applicable for laparoscopy. The miniaturization involves a) the reduction of joints and stem diameters (from the current size of 18mm to 10-12mm), and b) the small scale implementation of the joy-stick actuation mechanism on the handle. Furthermore, the actuation of tendons can also be performed through servo-controls for robotic applications as will be described in Ch.6 .

Chapter 4

AUTOMATED DEVICES

Generally, in most surgical procedures it is required to make incisions, and sometime to remove defective tissues (e.g. gall bladder removal). Thus, it is essential to perform accurate ligation of bleeding points, and re-approximate any incisions made during a surgical dissection, in order to complete the surgical procedure [75]. In laparoscopy, the tissue re-approximation and ligation is achieved primarily by different techniques of suturing (e.g. single stitches, or multi-running stitches), and knotting (e.g. square knots, or slip knots)[75][85]. In some cases special tools such as staplers, clips, and ring applicators are used [21][80].

The suturing and knotting are performed by a pair of needle drivers[1], and the surgical needle. However, suturing and knotting are considered some of the most difficult and time-consuming tasks of surgery[2]. These results were obtained based on motion/time study of the actual surgery, and a survey of 78 surgeons[13]. In summary, the level of difficulty and time needed for suturing and knotting are due to the following factors:

I) **Numerous movements required for each subtask:** There are a total of 11 subtasks for the suturing and knotting tasks. Each subtask involves several movements of the tool in order to be performed (i.e. for suturing 29, knotting 10, and cutting suture 5, with a total of 44 movements[13] for each stitch, see Table 4.1).

II) **Required internal dexterity:** Most of the movements require a specific orientation of the tool in order to be performed successfully

[1] i.e. especially designed graspers for manipulation of the needle and suture

[2] These tasks take between 3.5 to 6 minutes to be performed for each single stitch.

(e.g. grasping the needle, or piercing the needle into the tissue). This is especially difficult with the current rigid stem graspers which require a lot of time and effort (e.g. to manipulate the needle until it has the proper orientation toward the tissue).

Dexterous graspers with the flexible stem, described in the previous section, could provide more dexterity to perform the suturing and knotting tasks. However, the sheer high number of movements in these tasks still makes them very time consuming and tedious to perform. The difficulty of suturing in laparoscopy arises from the fact that surgeons, based on their past experience, are used to perform these tasks almost with the same techniques, and manual movements, as used in open surgery. In laparoscopy, they are faced with using two long graspers (instead of free hand), indirect vision, and having no haptic force feedback from the surgical site[Ch.1].

The great difficulty of performing such a routine task motivated us to develop special purpose devices that can perform them semi-automatically. For example, suturing and knotting tasks are carried out primarily through controlled manual movement of the needle. The objective of the design is to develop a suturing device which can generate a set of movements for the needle automatically. The surgeon simply guides the device for passing the suturing thread through the tissue *faster*, with much more *ease*, and *dexterity*. However, to determine the basic requirements of such a development, first we have to study the details of subtasks[13] involved in the manual suturing in Table 4.1:

Table 4.1. Duration of suturing subtasks in laparoscopy.

Subtasks	No. of movements	Ave. duration (sec): Novice	Expert
1- Position needle	3	103	51
2- Bite tissue	4	15	20
3- Pull needle thru	5	25	17
4- Re-position needle	4	35	13
5- Re-bite tissue	4	22	15
6- Re-pull needle thru	5	23	13
7- Pull suture thru	4	32	24
Total	29	255	153

By combining similar tasks in the above table, the subtasks can be summarized in the following categories:

Table 4.2. Categories of subtasks in suturing task.

Categories	Subtasks	% of total time
I) Capturing and orienting the needle	1 and 4	40-60%
II) Penetrating Tissue	2 and 5	15-25%
III) Needle re-capturing	3 and 6	15-20%

From the above, it is evident that : 1) almost 50% of the time is spent to capture and orient the needle to a specific orientation, 2) secure the grasp on the needle and penetrate the tissue to some desired orientation, which takes about 20% of the total time, and 3) re-capturing the emerging needle from the other side of tissue takes another 20% of the time.

The above results indicate that the suturing device must have the following functional features in order to be faster, and easier to perform the tasks compared to the manual suturing.

1) **Fixed needle :** The needle should have some specific *fixed position* and *orientation* on the device initially, so half the total time would not be lost for its capturing and orienting.

2) **Controlled penetrating motion :** The device should also provide the penetrating movement of the needle in the desired trajectory.

3) **Recapturing mechanism :** The device has to recapture the needle as it emerges from the other side of tissue, and provide the initial fixed orientation of the needle for the next cycle of suturing.

These are a very demanding set of requirements for a small mechanism with the diameter of 5-10mm to operate inside the body. There exist several proposed types of designs in the literature [58] [59][63] [64]. Among these designs, those which were implemented successfully are basically related to a single type of design based on *reciprocating actuation*. For example, Neisius and Melzer developed the *linear reciprocating* jaws (Fig.4.1a) where a needle is transfered and intermittently locked between the two jaws pneumatically. The needle has a central cross bore for the thread which is passed through the tissue in each actuation cycle. They modified the design to another more compact version with pneumatically actuated *rotary* jaws similar to the design of a grasper (Fig.4.1b). Similar design concepts have been employed by U.S. Surgical in the commercially available device called *Auto-Suture*[91] where

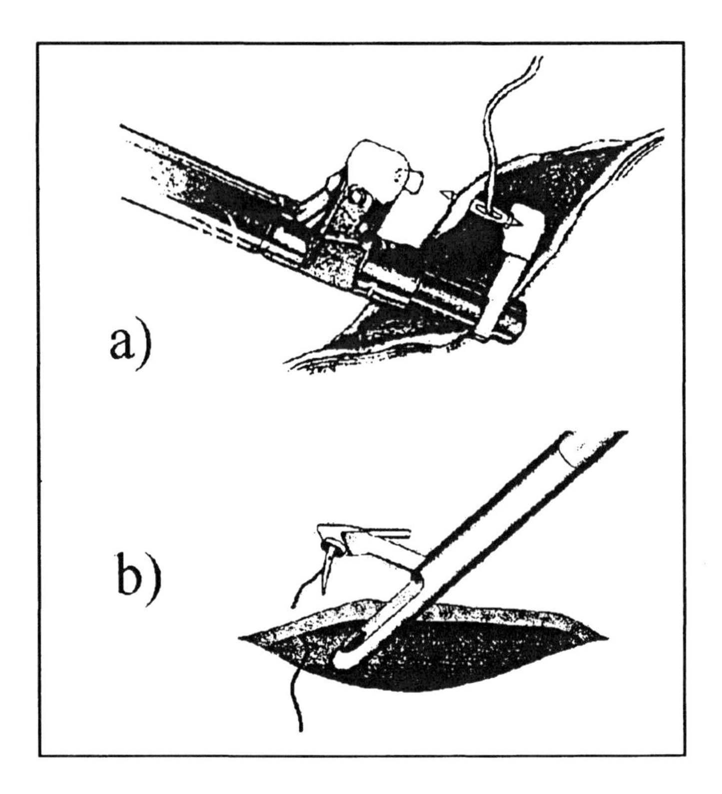

Figure 4.1. Suturing device with reciprocating jaws and needle.

actuation is done manually. Another version of reciprocating suturing devices is proposed, by Laurus Medical Corporation[52], which uses a small "shuttle needle ", that passes through the tissue by an arc-shaped carrier to a capturing port (Fig.4.2) .

The above mentioned developments, based on reciprocation of needles, satisfy all the three requirements mentioned above. However, they face some draw backs due to reciprocating motion that can be stated as :

a) Limits on the thickness of the tissue to be sutured. This is due to the limitation on the length of the stroke.

b) Possibility of tissue damage due to reciprocating motion of jaws when they are closed.

c) Possibility of failure in recapturing the needle by the other jaw due to lateral suturing forces.

d) In the case of pneumatic actuation, there would be lack of control on the movement/force of the needle while penetrating the tissue.

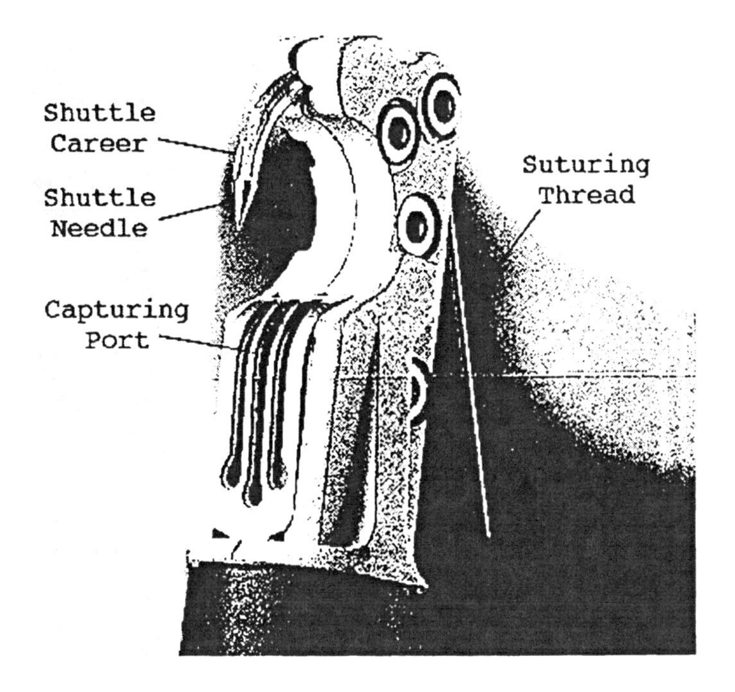

Figure 4.2. Suturing device with reciprocating shuttle needle.

To avoid these short-comings another class of suturing device based on *continuous circular motion* (CCM) with an arc shaped needle is studied in the following section.

1. NEW SUTURING DEVICE WITH CCM DESIGN

Arc shaped needles are the standard and the most common type of needle used in surgery[75]. This is due to the fact that the needle can penetrate and exit the tissue in one stroke of circular motion, without the need to re-orient the needle in order to exit the tissue. In this research, based on the existing manual suturing technique that surgeons are quite familiar with, another class of suturing device is studied and prototyped (Fig.4.3 to 4.7) [24][32]. This semi-automated suturing device for laparoscopy provides the surgeon with an ideal continuous suturing motion similar to the manual stitching used in open surgery. The primary challenges of this design and development are: a) the guidance tracks for the needle, and b) the actuation mechanism of the needle around the circular path, which are described further in the followings:

a) **Guiding Tracks :** The circular arcs of both the needle and the guiding tracks must be greater than 180° (by at least a safe margin of 45° – 60°), so the tip of needle would re-enter the tracks again after its penetration of the tissue is accomplished (Fig.4.5b)[24]. On the other hand, if the opening of the suturing head tracks is less than 120°, there may not be sufficient space for placing the tissue into the head. Hence, an arc angle of 240° both for the needle and guiding tracks was selected to ensure that at any position of needle, at least half of the length of the needle is guided and actuated on the tracks, while the other half is engaged in suturing.

The structure of tracks is shown in cross-sectional view in Fig.4.3b, which consists of two circular guiding plates each mounted on the top and bottom frames of the suturing device. The function of the guiding plates are: a) to keep the needle securely behind the guiding plates so it does not disengage from the head, b) to provide the radial support for the needle so the belt can exert radial force on it, which in turn causes tangential actuation by the friction force, c) the slit between the two plates acts as the guiding track for the circular cross section of the needle, and d) the slit provides an opening where the suturing thread can be pulled out after each cycle of the needle around the tracks (Fig.4.3b). There are also two additional top and bottom supporting plates (Fig.4.3b) which prevent the needle from any movements and misalignments in the normal direction to the plane of the circular arc.

b) **Actuation Mechanism :** The actuation of the needle is provided by a friction belt which due to its tension, snugs around the needle tightly for an angular contact of 240° (Fig.4.3a)[24]. This is obtained by a series of 5 guiding rollers which guide the belt around the track as well as pressing the belt further to the needle. Type of the belt and its method of actuation by frictional traction of the needle around the path are further discussed in the following section.

2. FRICTION ANALYSIS OF THE BELT MECHANISM

Type and size synthesis of the belt are the crucial design steps since it plays a central roll in guidance and actuation. In this regard, the friction belt, as the simplest type of belt, is initially studied in this section. This flat belt, which passes through the guiding tracks and several idlers, also wraps around the drive pulley (Fig.4.3a). The primary objective in this section is to verify the possibility of actuating the belt around the path

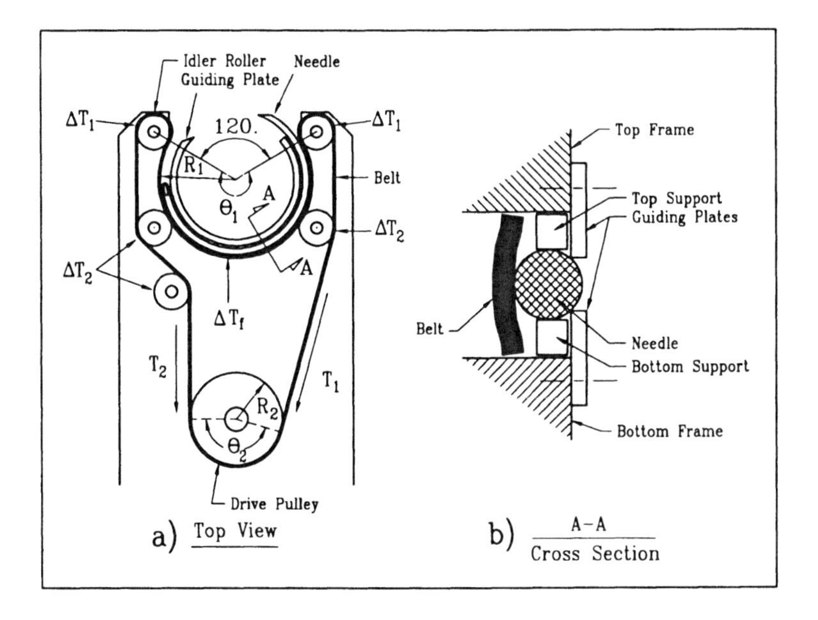

Figure 4.3. Suturing device with circulating needle.

by friction traction of the drive pulley. The equation for tension in a flat belt actuated by a frictional drive pulley[19] can be written as:

$$T_2 = T_1 e^{-\mu\theta} \tag{4.1}$$

where T_1 and T_2 are the tension before and after the drive pulley with the Coulomb frictional coefficient μ, and θ being the wrap angle of the belt around the pulley. A similar equation can be used to estimate the tension of the belt while wrapping around the 240° arc of the track. The only difference here is the use of the dynamic coefficient of friction μ_d due to the relative motion of the belt and needle with respect to the stationary track.

In order for the pulley to be able to actuate the belt without slippage, the tension difference of belt before and after the pulley (T_1 and T_2 respectively) must be greater than the resisting forces in the loop, that can be written as:

$$T_1 - T_2 > \Delta T_f + 2\Delta T_1 + 3\Delta T_2 \tag{4.2}$$

where ΔT_f is the incremental increase in tension due to friction between the belt and tracks, and ΔT_1 and ΔT_2 are the frictional resistance of idlers (Fig.4.3a). To simplify the above inequality, the unknown parameters ΔT_1 and ΔT_2 can be removed to obtain:

$$T_1 - T_2 >> \Delta T_f \tag{4.3}$$

Using Eq. (4.1) we can also write :

$$T_1 - T_2 = T_1(1 - e^{-\mu_2\theta_2})$$
$$\Delta T_f = T_1(1 - e^{-\mu_1\theta_1})$$

Where μ_1, and θ_1 are the coefficient of friction and wrap-angle of the belt around the track, while μ_2, and θ_2 are same parameters of the belt around the drive pulley. By substituting the above equations in the inequality (4.3), and after simplification we get :

$$\mu_2\theta_2 >> \mu_1\theta_1 \tag{4.4}$$

From the previous section, the value of θ_1 was selected to be 240° in order the device to function. On the other hand, the values of μ_1 and μ_2 are not reliably known in the wet and lubricated conditions of surgical site, which causes their values to drop to low values in the range of 0.05 to 0.1[7]and vary significantly depending on the amount of lubrication caused by bodily fluids at the surgical site. Therefore, by substituting $\theta_1 = 240°$ in Eq. (4.4), and having the conservative assumption $\mu_1 = \mu_2 \approx 0.05$ would result:

$$\theta_2 >> 240° \tag{4.5}$$

Even by using extra idlers in order to maximize the contact angle (θ_2) of the belt around the drive pulley (close to 240°), still it is not possible to satisfy Eq. (4.5) and subsequently Eq. (4.2). This means that friction pulley can not be a practical solution despite some patented claims[10] for suturing devices with friction belt drives.

Therefore, the next design belt type would be the timing belt, which by positive engagement of the toothed belt with pulley provides sufficient actuation force without any slippage (Fig.4.4). The details of the transmission mechanism and related prototyping issues are described in the following section.

3. LARGE SCALE EXPERIMENTAL PROTOTYPE

The first experimental prototype was built with external diameter of 33mm, which is a scaled up version of laparoscopic size (by a factor of 3 compared to the acceptable size range of 10-12mm for laparoscopy). This enlarged prototype is for the purpose of studying the mechanism, as well as ' e proof-of-concept for the device functionality, while avoiding following problems of miniaturization :

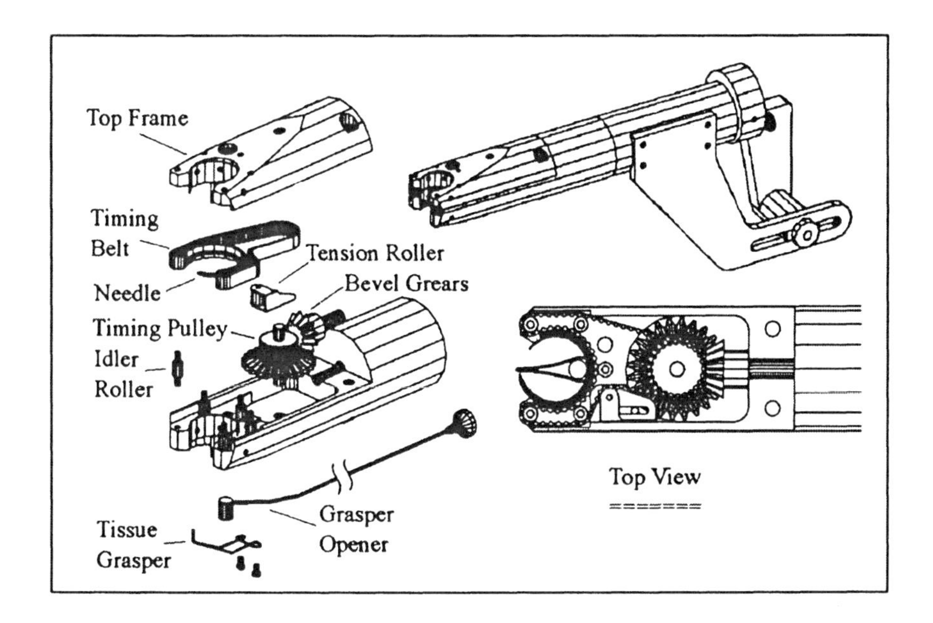

Figure 4.4. The design assembly of suturing device with circulating needle.

a) Avoiding high precision machining and fabrication which exceeds the available machine shop resources.

b) Avoiding miniature special parts, such as miniature timing belts, bevel gears, etc, by using larger standard parts already available off the shelf.

The exploded view and internal details of the prototype are shown in Fig.4.4 . The path of the timing belt and guiding tracks have the same configuration as shown in Fig.4.3 . The timing belt is a standard size (4.5mm wide, 1.2mm thick, with a tooth pitch of 2.07mm) made of polyurethane and reinforced with polyester cords[79]. The tension of the timing belt is adjusted by a movable "tension idler", which is secured in place on the main frame by a locking screw (Fig.4.4). The actuation of the belt is provided by the timing pulley, which is turned by a set of bevel gears. The rotary motion of the gears are transfered by a shaft which is connected to a hand wheel at the handle for manual actuation.

The additional design feature of the suturing device is related to the tissue grasper. This small grasper provides the required support for delicate and compliant tissues which are difficult to pierce by the needle without deflecting them away. This can be added to the device, and perform the suturing task much more effectively as shown in Fig.4.5a-c. The first step of suturing using the device would be to open the compliant

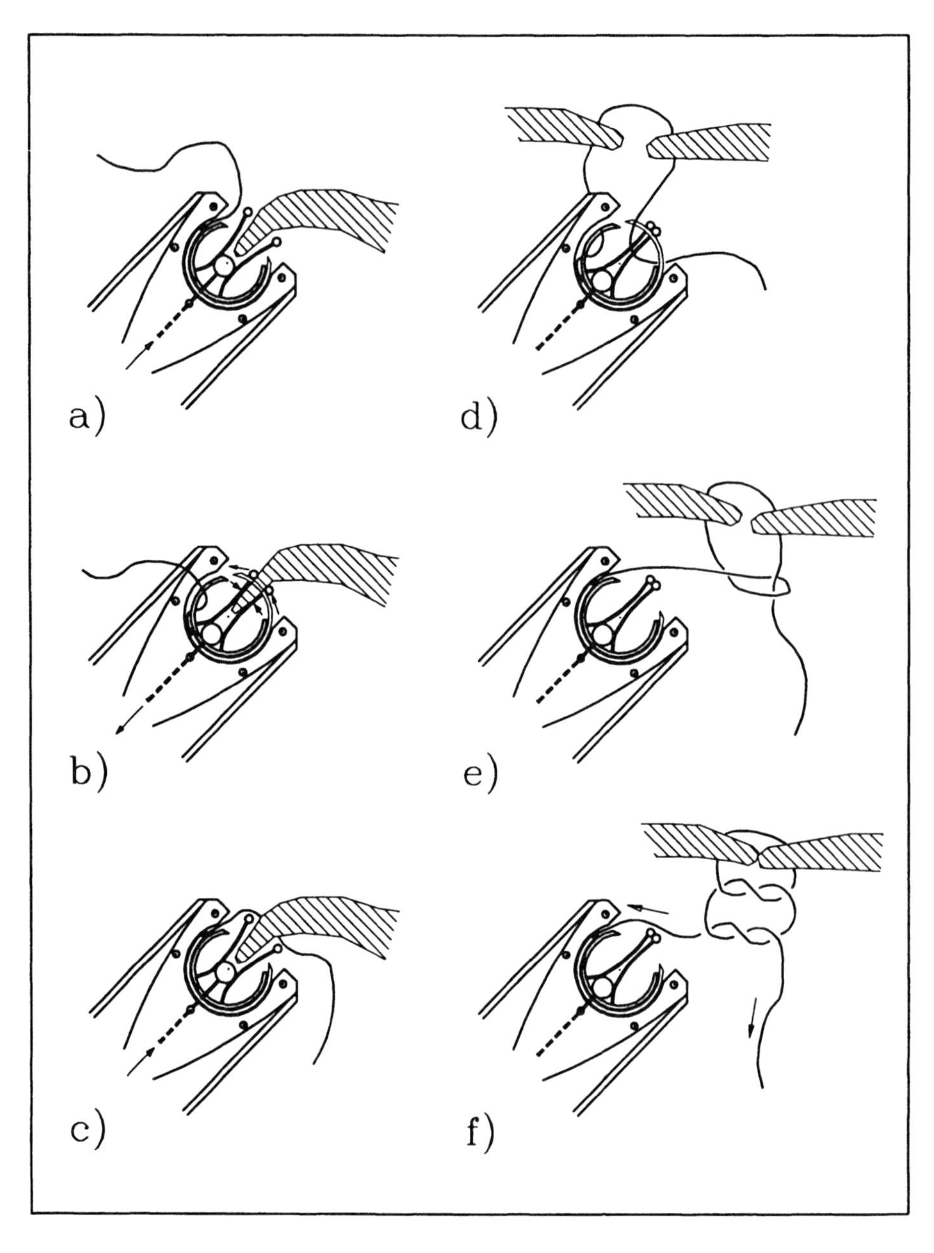

Figure 4.5. Different steps of suturing and knotting with the new device.

jaws of the grasper (Fig.4.5a) by pushing in the "grasper opener", and letting the tissue to get in between the open jaws. Then by closing the jaws, the tissue is secured, and held firmly in a fixed position with respect to the suturing head, while the needle can penetrate it (Fig.4.5b). The last step would be to open the grasper and release the tissue after the

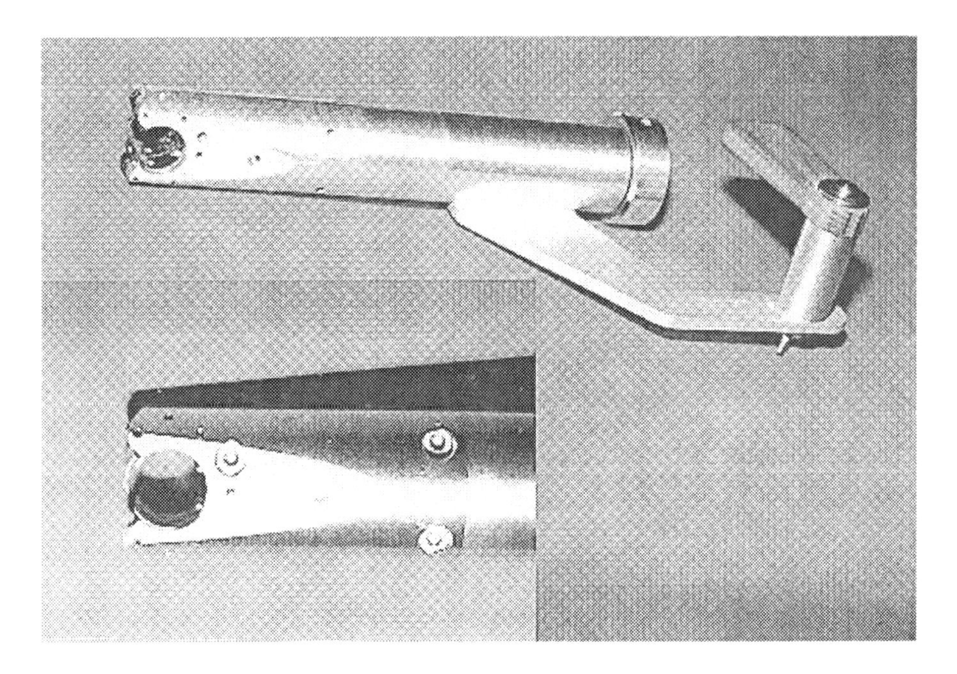

Figure 4.6. The first prototype of the suturing device.

suture is passed through by 360° rotation of needle (Fig.4.5c). Same can be performed to the other side of the tissue to be approximated (Fig.4.5d), and then knotting can be executed by looping the needle around the other end of suturing thread (Fig.4.5d, and Fig.4.5e), which creates a slip knot. By repeating same knotting procedure once more and pulling the two ends of the thread, a square knot can be formed, which can securely approximate and hold the two sides of tissue together.

With the enlarged prototype (Fig.4.6), it has been possible to perform both suturing and knotting tasks within one minute, with the least amount of effort, by experimenting on tissue-like medium (e.g. urethane foam). This encouraging result verified the functionality of the suturing device, compared to laborious manual technique (which takes on average 5-10 minutes to perform each suture and knot by two graspers[13]). This motivated us to move to the next level of experimental development of the actual-size prototyping of such a device.

4. MINIATURIZATION CHALLENGES

Considering the fact that the current laparoscopic tools and instruments are in the range of 5 to 12mm, for the next stage of prototyping and miniaturization it has been decided to work on the possibility of a 12mm version (Fig.4.7). This stage proved quite challenging, both in

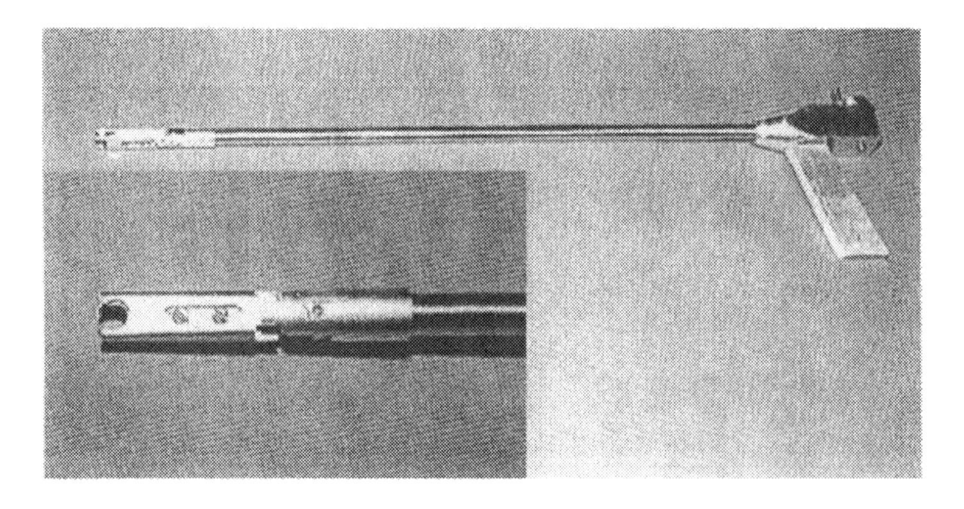

Figure 4.7. The miniaturized prototype for laparoscopy.

terms of precision machining, as well as obtaining suppliers for special parts such as timing belts or bevel gears.

It has been possible to address partially the high precision machining problems, by obtaining funding and purchasing a small precision turning/milling machine.

The bevel gear transmission was replaced by the smallest size of available timing belts (i.e. 3mm wide, and 1.2mm thick) to transfer rotary motion from the handle to the miniaturized suturing head (Fig.4.8). However, the transmission belt could not be used to actuate the needle directly due to its high thickness (1.2mm), as well as its requirement for the minimum diameter of its idler ($> 5mm$). Hence, two pulleys are fixed together (on a common shaft) to transfer the rotational motion from the transmission belt to another much thinner belt (i.e. 0.4mm thick) called the actuation belt (Fig.4.8) for actuation of the needle.

Several types of timing belts have been studied as candidates for the actuation belt. For example, metallic timing belts were considered as a promising alternative, since they are much thinner than plastic belts. However, due to the high stiffness of steel belts, the minimum bending diameter around idlers is limited to:

$$d \geq 200t \tag{4.6}$$

In addition, the suturing head diameter D is subject to the following constraint:

$$D \geq w + 2(d + 2t) \tag{4.7}$$

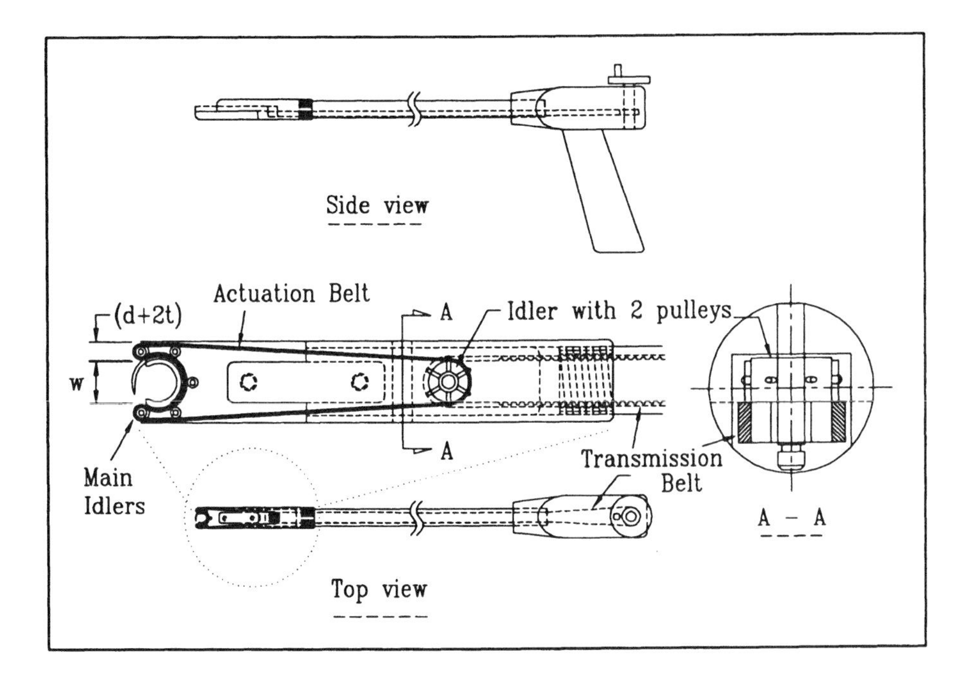

Figure 4.8. The design of miniaturized prototype.

Where w is the width of opening on the suturing head for the tissue to be sutured (Fig.4.8). The minimum acceptable limit of w for the suturing head with diameter $D = 12mm$ is considered to be in the range of $w \geq 6mm$. Parameters $(d + 2t)$ represent the total diameter of the two main idlers (diameter d) and belt around them $(2t)$. By applying these values in Eq. (4.6) and (4.7) we obtain:

$12 \geq 6 + 404t \Longrightarrow t \leq 0.015mm$

This range of value for belt thickness is not viable for the metal belt, due to stress concentration at the engaged teeth, as well as the minimum belt thickness supplied by the manufacturer of such belts[9] starting from 0.07mm.

The next alternative was polyester flat belts with Neoprene coating [79]. It can be converted to timing belt by perforating the belt for our application. The promising aspect of this kind of belt is its relatively low thickness (0.4mm) and high flexibility. Thus the minimum bend diameter can be in the order of : $d \geq 5t$ for a limited operating life cycles. Substituting this constraint in Eq. (4.7) would result: $t \leq 0.43mm$ which is in the range of the actual belt thickness.

Based on the above, a second prototype with idlers of 2mm in diameter, and the polyester belt with 3mm width has been developed (Fig.4.7). However, the attempt to convert the flat belt to a timing belt,

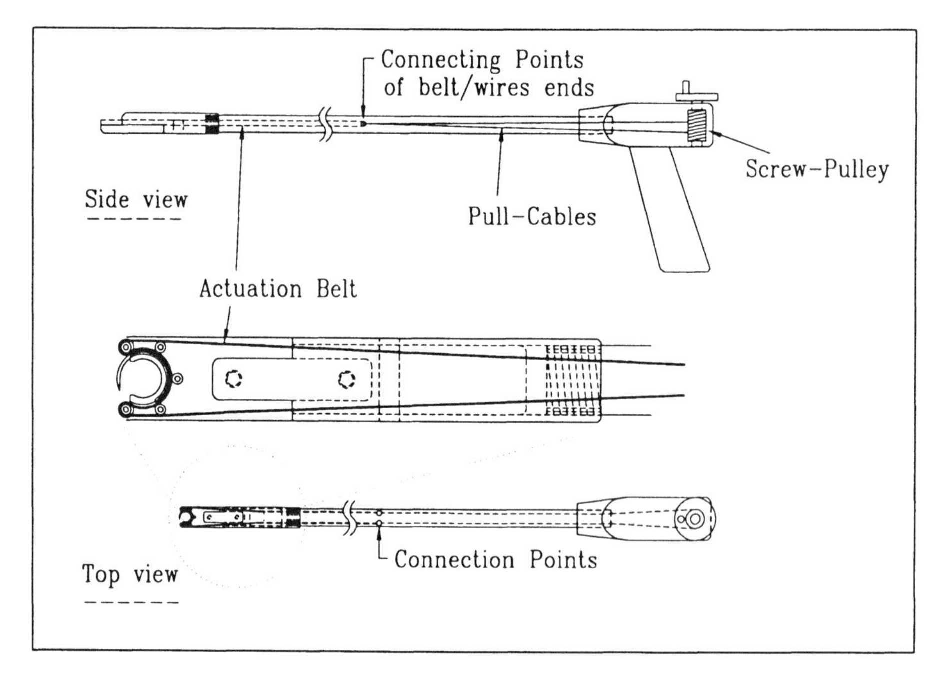

Figure 4.9. The design of miniaturized prototype with open end belt-drive.

by perforating it with 0.8mm holes at a pitch distance of 3.2mm, did not provide satisfactory results. The belt became mechanically too weak due to its small width and added perforations, which failed under operating tension in very limited numbers of cycles.

The next attempt was to use similar flat belt material (polyester) in an open-end configuration that the ends are attached to cable wires (0.3 mm thick). The wires actuate the belt by pulling its ends, and the wires in turn are actuated by a multi-revolution screw-pulley (Fig.4.9). The trade-off in this type of actuation is that, due to the open end configuration of the flat belt, the maximum number of revolutions of the needle is limited to the length of the belt (i.e. maximum of 8-10 revolutions for the design, compared to 4 revolutions required for tissue penetrations and square knotting of each stitch). This approach resulted in successful actuation of the needle by the belt around the track. However, this could not be developed to a working prototype for clinical trial, due to the high level of friction still present between the belt and the tracks. This makes the actuation difficult, which requires high forces combined with repetitive cloggings. Further development of the miniaturized suturing device requires a suitable flat belt material with sufficient flexibility and strength. An example of such material would be high tensile nylon, reinforced with longitudinal glass fibers, which requires to be manufactured as special order by related manufacturers for the final development of the suturing device.

Chapter 5

FORCE REFLECTING GRASPERS

Due to the physical barrier of the abdominal wall in laparoscopy, the operation is based on *remote manipulation.* Hence, in contrast to the open surgery, direct sensation of the surgical site and palpation is not possible. There have been attempts [16][35][70] to compensate for this lack of tactile sensing by using an *array of tactile sensors* that measures the pressure distribution (or small-scale shape distribution), and recreating this by using an *array of tactile displays* on the hand of surgeon. The design of tactile sensors is even more complicated if we want to incorporate sensations of temperature and vibration as part of the tactile sensing.

Another important missing sensory feedback is the sensation of the grasping force which is not reflected properly by laparoscopic forceps. Recent studies [83][82] indicates that the ratio of the grasping force to the handle force (which ideally must be constant and equal to the transmission ratio of the forceps from the grasper to the handle) varies greatly depending on the mechanical properties of the object to be squeezed. Also, other studies[41][40] show that forces at the handle, grasper, and the hand muscle while manipulating with laparoscopic forceps are significantly different from those when using conventional surgical forceps. The result is much less control over the grasping force at the surgical site by laparoscopic graspers. As a consequence, a number of injuries during laparoscopic procedures have been reported that usually do not occur during conventional surgeries.

In general, the grasping force at the tip of the laparoscopic grasper is sensed poorly at the handle due to the friction, backlash, and the stiffness[1] present in all the intermediate mechanical linkages. Especially, when manipulating delicate soft tissues, the required grasping force is very small, and its sensation is prone to be lost under the influence of the friction and backlash in all the linkages. In this case the force reflection to the handle is poor, and there exists the possibility of damaging delicate tissues due to the lack of proper force reflection to the hand of the surgeon.

All of the above drawbacks of the current state-of-the art, lead us to the following primary requirements as the motivation for new designs of graspers with force reflection:

Requirement I) To have *adjustable* force transmission between the handle and grasper, so that the surgeon can adjust the handle forces to higher levels compatible with his/her gripping force sensitivity. This should be accomplished while keeping forces at the grasper proportionally lower compatible with the tissue compliance.

Requirement II) To be able to monitor and limit the maximum level of grasping force, in order to prevent any possible tissue damage.

For any design to meet the above requirements successfully, it should provide sufficient bandwidth[2] in order to reflect and respond to the grasping forces which are dynamically changing. In the following sections, first some design concepts are studied which address the above requirements, and after synthesis, the control and bandwidth issues are discussed, followed by the experimental analysis.

1. DESIGN CONCEPTS

Generally, for a design to be applicable to laparoscopic graspers, it has to be compact and light. In this respect, the following four general classes of designs are considered as possible design concepts:

Class 1- The first requirement could be satisfied by designing a grasper with a *mechanical* variable ratio of transmission (i.e. r from point D to A, Fig. 5.1a), by simply moving the pivot point of the handle (i.e. point C, Fig. 5.1a, or by changing length of BC by moving B), so the overall transmission ratio r of the grasper can be adjusted. However with this design, the second design requirement can not be satisfied.

[1] Caused by the elastic deflection of all intermediate linkage members.

[2] The bandwidth of a device is defined as the maximum speed or frequency at which the device is capable of operating[18].

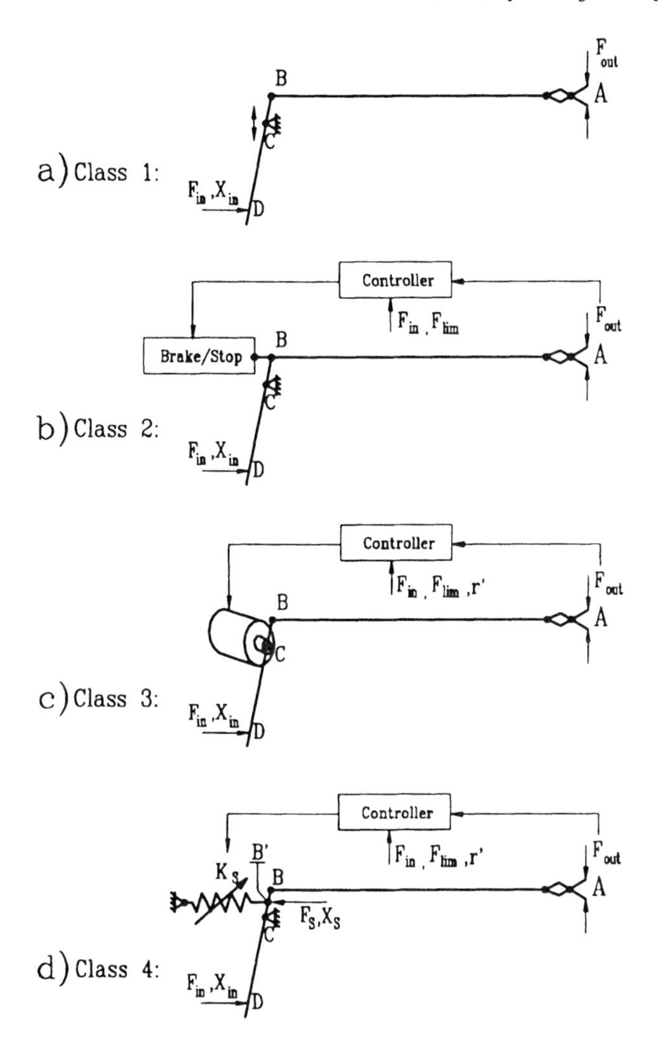

Figure 5.1. Four different classes of forceps design with adjustable grasping force.

Class 2- The second requirement could be satisfied by sensing the grasping force F_{out}, then comparing it with the desired maximum force limit F_{lim} to activate a brake, or to control a stop limit that prevents any further motion transmission from the handle to the grasper (Fig. 5.1b). However the first requirement of variable transmission ratio can not be achieved with this design.

Class 3- By simply using a high torque motor at joint C (Fig. 5.1c) as a direct drive, and sensing F_{in} and F_{out}, it is possible to have computed feedback control, so that both of the requirements can be satisfied.

Class 4- By using a "variable" or "tunable" spring whose stiffness K_s could be changed (or controlled), it is possible to distribute part of the input hand force F_{in} to the grasper (so that it satisfies Req.I and/or II), and absorb the remaining force through the tunable spring connected to intermediate linkages (Fig. 5.1d, with the transmission ratio $r_s := \frac{B'C}{DC} = \frac{X_s}{X_{in}}$). This design has the potential to address both requirements provided that a proper controller is incorporated into the design (described in Sec.4.2).

To meet both of the requirements, either Class 3 or 4 can be used individually, or a combination of Classes 1 and 2 can be used as the final design. The combination of Classes 1 and 2 would be far more difficult to implement (with two separate actuation and control systems for each class) and less feasible for successful operation than Classes 3 or 4 individually. Class 3 is the typical solution for tele-operation and force reflection[88]. However, this design may require a relatively bulky actuator to provide the required torque (e.g., even for 1.4 Nm (190 Oz-in) stalling torque, the size of DC motor would be approximately OD.70×120mm weighing 1.5Kg[3], and for a torque motor with 1.7Nm (230 Oz-in) peak torque, OD.100×40mm[4]). The current sheer size and weight of these direct drive systems makes them impractical to use for the application even if they meet the requirements. On the other hand, the tunable spring needs a relatively much smaller motor, and if it meets the requirements (as discussed in the next sections), then it would be a viable alternative for further analysis and development. In this chapter, the efforts are focused on Class 4 by using analytical methods, simulations, and experimental prototyping to evaluate this type of design.

2. TYPE SYNTHESIS OF TUNABLE SPRING

The tunable spring is the most important component in the design (Class 4), and its general requirements can be summarized in the followings:

A - The stiffness of spring must be variable in a range that at the lowest stiffness setting generates minimal resistance force at the handle to allow the surgeon to close the graspers jaws with minimum effort and force (e.g. 3-5 N [15]).

[3]MicroMo Electronics Inc., PM DC motor series GNM 4125.
[4]Servo System Co. Cat. No. 3730-134H-019.

B - The stiffness of the spring must be variable in a range that at the highest stiffness setting generates maximum stiffness at the handle, hence the surgeon would feel near absolute rigidity at the handle (e.g. as high as 100 N/mm).

C - The spring must not plastically deform in the full range of stiffness variation under the highest force generated by the surgeon at the handle (e.g. maximum 50 N [15]).

D - The actuation of the tunable spring should not interfere with the movements of the grasper, which is controlled from the handle only by the hand movements of the surgeon. Therefore, the connecting point of the spring to the linkages (i.e. point B', Fig.5.7) should not move due to the actuation of the spring (when the spring is not loaded). The purpose of the spring actuation is only to change/control its stiffness K_s. Hence, the force generated by the spring F_s should always remain as the product of its stiffness and the displacement which is generated only by the displacement of the handle (i.e. $X_s = r_s X_{in} => F_s = K_s X_s = K_s r_s X_{in}$, Fig.5.8).

Considering the above requirements, there are numerous design possibilities for tunable springs. For example, a novel design of tunable spring[51] uses two non-linear springs, with different stiffness characteristics, that are connected to each other in series. This design can not be used here, since the range of stiffness is not wide enough[51] to satisfy requirements **A**, and **B** simultaneously. Also, requirement **D** can not be fulfilled either, since the connecting point in the middle of the two springs moves as they are actuated[51], causing the grasper and handle to have undesirable movements.

There is another class of tunable spring[17] whose stiffness is varied by changing the effective length of the spring from the total available length. This class is considered in this application due to its wide range of stiffness which satisfies requirements **A**, and **B**. Furthermore, only straight leaf spring is considered here, since the movement of the supporting points in straight leaf springs can be achieved by simple linear motion. This makes it a very suitable candidate for the variable stiffness spring designs. While satisfying all of the above requirements, it is easier to implement in comparison with more complicated spring shapes (e.g. closed loop, spiral, or helical springs).

For the type synthesis of the straight leaf spring, three types of supports are considered (Fig. 5.2):

Type 1- In this case, the leaf spring is supported only at two points (B) with equal distances of X from the center of the spring (Fig. 5.2a).

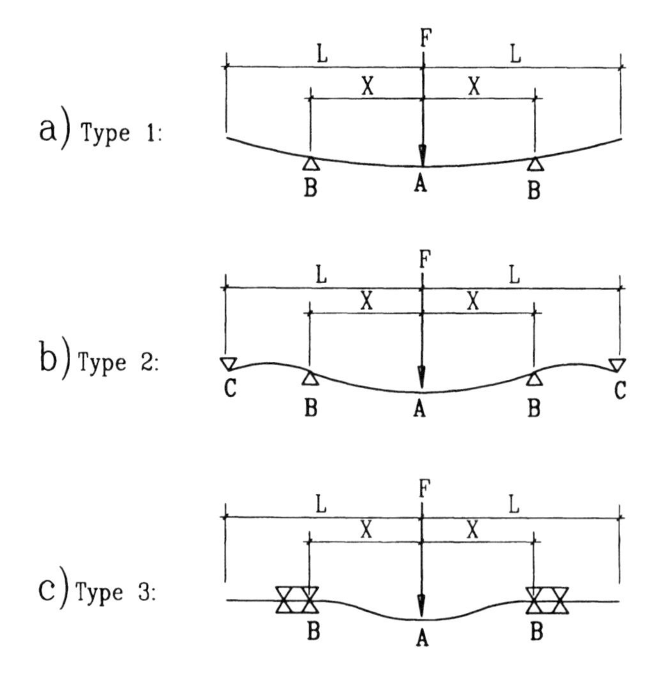

Figure 5.2. Three types of tunable springs using leaf springs.

The supporting points can prevent the spring from vertical deflection only.

Type 2- As shown in Fig. 5.2b, this kind of support is similar to *Type.1*, but the end points of the spring are also constrained to have zero deflection in Y direction.

Type 3- In this type (Fig. 5.2c), the supporting points are considered as guiding slits that keep both the deflection and the slope of the spring at distance X equal to zero.

In the next section, stiffness and bending analysis is carried out to evaluate the best type of support as well as to obtain mathematical models of the stiffness of the spring and the corresponding bending moments for further design optimization.

2.1 STIFFNESS AND BENDING ANALYSIS

Type 1 (Fig. 5.2a) is basically a two-point supported beam such that its stiffness K_1, and the maximum bending moment M_1^{max}, for small deflections are known[7] to be:

$$K_1 = \frac{6EI}{X^3} \tag{5.1}$$

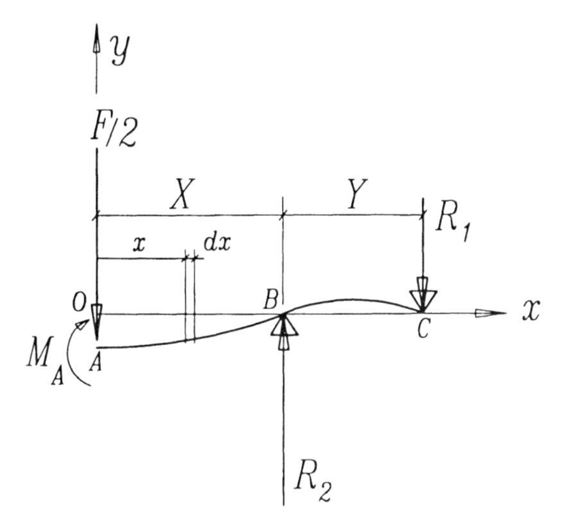

Figure 5.3. Loads on the symmetrical half of leaf spring.

$$M_1^{max} = \frac{FX}{2} \tag{5.2}$$

Where E is the module of elasticity, and $I = bt^3/12$ is the moment of inertia of the spring for the rectangular cross section with thickness t, and width b.

The other two types of design (Fig. 5.2b, and c) can be analyzed by the following general formulation. It is assumed that the flexible leaf spring is supported at two points (i.e. points B and C) on each side at distances of X and Y as shown in Fig. 5.3 . Assuming the frictional forces at these points are negligible, the equilibrium equations of forces and moments acting on the spring would be:

$$\sum \mathbf{F_y} = R_1 - R_2 - \tfrac{F}{2} = 0$$
$$\sum \mathbf{M_o} = -M_A + R_1 X - R_2(X+Y) = 0$$

By eliminating R_1 in the above equations: $M_A = \frac{F}{2}X - R_2 Y$, which is used in the equation of bending moment of the spring: $M(x) = M_A - \frac{F}{2}x$. That provides the following bending equation:

$$\frac{d^2\delta}{dx^2} = \frac{M(x)}{EI} = (\frac{F}{2}X - R_2 Y - \frac{F}{2}x)/EI$$

Solving the above for the boundary conditions (i.e. zero deflections at points B, and C, and zero slope at point A), it yields the following solution for the deflection of mid-point A:

$$\delta = \frac{FX^2(X+Y)^2}{24EI(X+Y/2)}$$

Solving for the stiffness K as the ratio of $\frac{F}{\delta}$ provides:

$$K = \frac{F}{\delta} = \frac{24EI(X+Y/2)}{X^2(X+Y)^2} \tag{5.3}$$

And the maximum bending moment of spring happens at point A and is:

$$M^{max} = \frac{F}{6}\left(\frac{3X^2+3XY+Y^2}{2X+Y}\right) \tag{5.4}$$

For Type 2, as a special case: $Y = L - X$, so equations (5.3) and (5.4) converts to:

$$K_2 = \frac{12EI}{X^2L^2}(X+L) \tag{5.5}$$

$$M_2^{max} = \frac{F}{6}\left(X + \frac{L^2}{X+L}\right) \tag{5.6}$$

While for Type 3, Y can be considered small and approximated as zero, hence equations (5.3) and (5.4) converts to:

$$K_3 = \frac{24EI}{X^3} \tag{5.7}$$

$$M_3^{max} = \frac{FX}{4} \tag{5.8}$$

Based on the above analysis, in order to select the best type of support, we have two design considerations: a) To have the widest stiffness range as a function of X/L. This will provide the smallest spring size as well as a fast response for the spring (due to the shorter traveling distance of the supports for tuning the spring in order to obtain the required stiffness). b) The maximum bending moment observed by the spring for the same load F should be the lowest, since the elastic limit of the spring is directly proportional to the maximum amount of bending moment (i.e. $\frac{MC}{I} < \sigma_y$, as yield stress).

To compare the three types, the stiffness K (Eq.5.1, 5.5, and 5.7) and the maximum bending moment M^{max} (Eq.5.2, 5.6, and 5.8) of all three types of springs are plotted (Fig.5.4a, and Fig.5.4b respectively) against the ratio of effective length over total length (i.e. X/L), while size, material properties, and applied force F are kept the same (i.e. $I = 3.38mm^4, L = 50mm, E = 210GPa$, and $F = 1000N$). It is evident from Fig. 5.4a and Fig. 5.4b that the spring design Type 3 has the

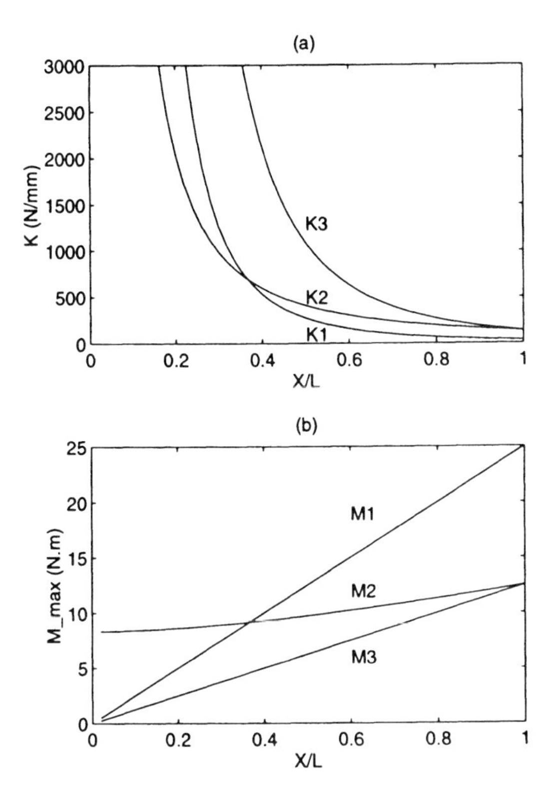

Figure 5.4. Stiffness K and bending moment M vs. X/L.

highest stiffness range (to meet requirements **A** and **B**), as well as the *lowest maximum bending moment* (providing highest flexibility before any undesirable plastic deformation of the spring). This makes Type 3 the best design of support for tunable leaf springs.

The above analysis and mathematical models for stiffness were based on the assumption of small deflection of the spring and no frictional forces at the supporting points. Hence, to verify the validity of the stiffness model (i.e. Eq.5.7), finite element method (FEM) is used. The finite element model is based on a 2D analysis by using 4-node brick elements (i.e. Solid42 of ANSYS software package) for modeling the leaf spring, and non-linear contact elements (i.e. Contac26, ANSYS) for modeling the friction at supporting points (Fig. 5.5). The size of each brick element is selected to be as fine as $0.2 \times 0.5mm$ for the leaf spring.

The finite element results for large deflections with friction at supporting points (assuming $\mu = 0.25$, shown with '+' sign in Fig. 5.6), and without friction (with 'x' sign) are shown in Fig. 5.6. The plot shows close agreement between the stiffness mathematical model (i.e. Eq.5.7,

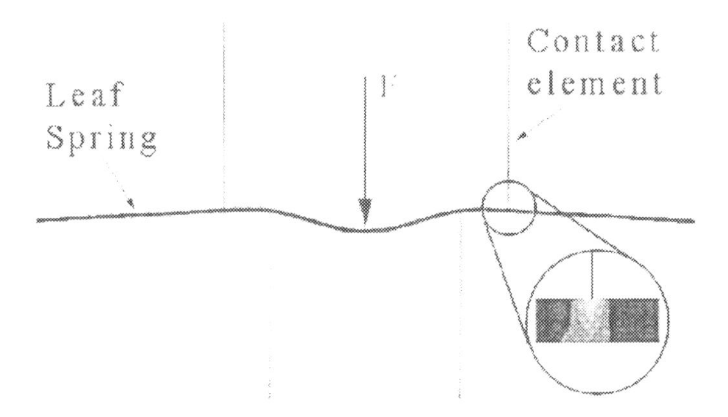

Figure 5.5. The FE model of deflected leaf spring under load supported by contact frictional elements.

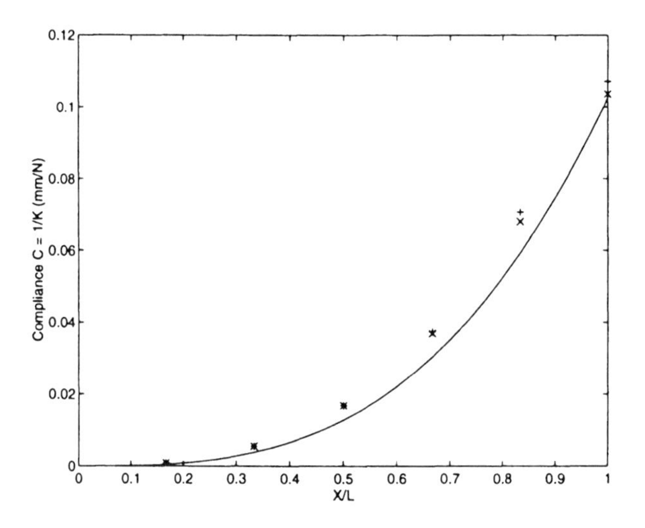

Figure 5.6. Compliance C vs. effective length ratio X/L .

shown as the solid line curve, Fig. 5.6) and the finite element results for both cases (with errors in the range of 0 to 15%).

In the following, the stiffness equation (5.7) is used in the closed loop control model (Sec. 4.2), as well as, for size synthesis and optimization of the design in the next section. Since Type 3 is the only spring type considered in the remaining of this chapter, then the stiffness of this type is referred as K_s, the stiffness of the spring, instead of K_3.

3. SIZE SYNTHESIS OF TUNABLE SPRING

The size synthesis of the tunable spring is carried out by optimization of the design variables, based on constraints and the objective function defined as:

- **Design Variables:** L (= half of spring's total length, Fig. 5.2c), b (width), t (thickness of the spring), and r_s as the transmission ratio from the handle to the spring.

- **Flexibility Constraint:** Based on requirement **A**, the spring with maximum effective length (i.e. $X = L$) should have a low stiffness so that it creates relatively small reaction forces at the handle (i.e. $F_{in}^{min} \leq 5N$, for the maximum displacement of the handle X_{in}^{max}). Also based on the spring force $F_s^{min} = K_s X_s^{max}$, and Eq.5.7 when $X = L$, we obtain:

$$F_s^{min} = (\frac{24EI}{L^3})X_s^{max} \tag{5.9}$$

  On the other hand due to transmission ratio r_s from handle to the spring, when the grasping force $F_{out} \approx 0$, we have:

  $F_s^{min} \leq F_{in}^{min}/r_s$, and $X_s^{max} = r_s X_{in}^{max}$. After substituting F_s^{min}, X_s^{max} in Eq.5.9, and rearranging for L, it provides the following constraint:

$$L \geq (2E\frac{X_{in}^{max}}{F_{in}^{min}})^{\frac{1}{3}}(b)^{\frac{1}{3}}(r_s)^{\frac{2}{3}}t \tag{5.10}$$

- **Elasticity Constraint:** Based on requirement **C**, in order to avoid any plastic deformation of the spring, the maximum bending stress σ^{max} must be less than the allowable stress (which is the yield stress σ_y divided by a safety factor N):

$$\sigma^{max} = \frac{Mc}{I} = \frac{M_3^{max}(t/2)}{bt^3/12} \leq \sigma_y/N$$

  M_3^{max} is obtained from Eq.5.8, and by substituting in it: $X = (24EIX_s^{max}/F_s^{max})^{\frac{1}{3}}$ from Eq.5.7, we convert the above equation to the following inequality:

$$\frac{3F_s^{max}(24EIX_s^{max}/F_s^{max})^{\frac{1}{3}}}{2bt^2} \leq \frac{\sigma_y}{N}$$

  Replacing $F_s^{max} = F_{in}^{max}/r_s$, $X_s^{max} = r_s X_{in}^{max}$, and rearranging for r_s provides us with the following constraint:

$$r_s \geq \frac{27E(F_{in}^{max})^2 X_{in}^{max} N^3}{4b^2t^3\sigma_y^3} \tag{5.11}$$

- **Strength Constraint:** The strength of joints and the stiffness of intermediate connecting links put an upper bound constraint on the maximum allowable spring force (e.g. in this case it is assumed that: $F_s^{lim} \leq 1000N$). On the other hand, $F_{in} = F_s r_s + F_{out} r$, or $r_s \geq F_{in}/F_s$, which creates the following constraint on r_s:

$$r_s \geq \frac{F_{in}^{max}}{F_s^{lim}} \tag{5.12}$$

- **Size limits:** For the solution to be in a genuine practical range compatible with size of the handle, the size variables such as b and t have to be bounded to the range which is practical to implement such as:

$$0 < b \leq 12.5mm, 0 < t \leq 6.0mm \tag{5.13}$$

- **Objective Function:** In order to minimize the size of leaf spring L, we can re-write the flexibility constraint (5.10) as:

$$MIN : L = (2E\frac{X_{in}^{max}}{F_{in}^{min}})^{\frac{1}{3}}(b)^{\frac{1}{3}}(r_s)^{\frac{2}{3}}t \tag{5.14}$$

- **Spring Material:** The spring parameters E, and σ_y have definitive influence on the optimized solution. The following spring materials with their related parameters [6] are considered for solutions of the size synthesis:

Table 5.1. The design parameters of different spring material.

No.	Spring Material	$\sigma_y(MPa)$	$E(GPa)$
1	Spring steel (SAE 1074)	1050	210
2	Si-Mn steel (SAE 9260)	1500	210
3	Cr-Si steel (SAE 9254)	1600	210
4	Nickel-Silver	665	112
5	Silicon-Bronze	600	105
6	Beryllium-Copper	1250	127

Numerically solving (by using MATLAB Optimization Toolbox) the above objective function (5.14), subject to the constraints (5.11), (5.12), (5.13), for different materials of Table 5.1, and by selecting the safety factor N=1.35 (to keep bending stresses below %75 of the yield stress), the results of Table 5.2 are obtained.

Table 5.2. The optimum design variables based on different spring material.

No.	Spring Material	$L(mm)$	$b(mm)$	$t(mm)$	r_s
1	Spring steel	76.2	12.5	2.3	0.05
2	Si-Mn steel	53.4	12.5	1.6	0.05
3	Cr-Si steel	50.0	12.5	1.5	0.05
4	Nickel Silver	79.2	12.5	2.9	0.05
5	Silicon Bronze	84.0	12.5	3.2	0.05
6	Beryllium Copper	45.0	12.5	1.6	0.05

From Table 5.2 it is evident that, the optimum material for this application is Beryllium-Copper with the highest yield strain ($\epsilon_y = \sigma_y/E = 9.8 \times 10^{-3}$), and the optimum design variables of : L= 45.0mm, b=12.5mm, t=1.6mm, and r_s=0.05 which provides the shortest spring length.

4. DESIGN INTEGRATION

The next objective is to integrate the spring and its actuation mechanism into the design of the grasper. The integration steps of the design consist of: a) the design of the actuation mechanism for the tunable spring, and b) the design of the controller, which are described in the following sections.

4.1 THE ACTUATION MECHANISM

The linear motion of supporting points at the two ends of the tunable spring can be generated for example by a lead screw mechanism coupled to pulleys and a motor (Fig. 5.7). The lead screw is divided into two equal lengths of left and right handed screws, which drives the connected nuts (as the supporting points of the spring) in a linear path.

The force f (exerted by the nuts, in longitudinal direction of X, to the spring on each side, Fig. 5.7) is the sum of: a) the friction force $f_f = \frac{\mu F_s}{2}$, and b) the actuation force f_a required to make the spring to comply to the new location of supporting points. Therefore $f = f_f \pm f_a$, and f_a would be :

$$f_a = \pm(f - f_f) = \pm(f - \mu F_s/2) \tag{5.15}$$

Neglecting frictional energy losses, and based on the principle of conservation of energy, the actuation energy $f_a(2\Delta X)$ (that $2\Delta X$ is the total of incremental displacement of the two nuts when the shaft rotates

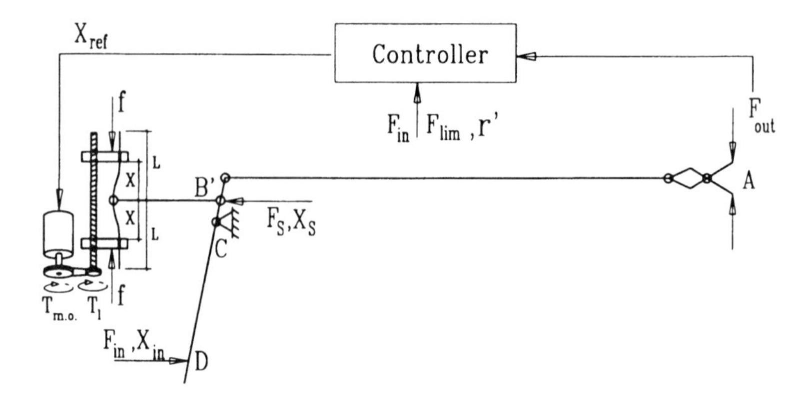

Figure 5.7. The force reflecting forceps with tunable leaf spring design.

incrementally) must be equal to the change in the deflection of spring $\Delta\delta$ multiplied by the applied force to the spring F_s:

$$f_a(2\Delta X) = F_s(\Delta\delta) \tag{5.16}$$

Also by differentiating the deflection equation $\delta = \frac{F_s}{K_s} = \frac{F_s X^3}{24EI}$ (by using Eq.5.7 for K_s), to obtain $\Delta\delta$ as:

$$\Delta\delta = \frac{3F_s X^2 \Delta X}{24EI} \tag{5.17}$$

Replacing (5.15) and (5.17) in (5.16) provides :

$$f = \pm\frac{F_s^2 X^2}{8EI} + \frac{\mu F_s}{2} \tag{5.18}$$

The torque required by the lead screw T_l to generate the thrust force f at each of the two nuts is known to be :

$$T_l = \frac{d(2f)}{2}\left[\frac{\pi d\mu \pm l\cos\theta}{\pi d\cos\theta \mp \mu l}\right] \tag{5.19}$$

Where d, l, and θ are the diameter, lead, and thread angle of the lead screw respectively, and μ the coefficient of friction. The upper signs correspond to the nuts' movement toward each other, and the lower signs to the nuts' movement away from each other. Replacing (5.18) in (5.19) and assuming $\mu l \approx 0$ (since $\mu l << \pi d\cos\theta$) provides the required torque to actuate the lead screw as :

$$T_l = \frac{d.F_s}{2}\left(\mu \pm \frac{F_s X^2}{4EI}\right)\left(\frac{\mu}{\cos\theta} \pm \frac{l}{\pi d}\right) \tag{5.20}$$

Hence the output torque of motor $T_{m.o.}$ after the reduction ratio of pulleys r_p would be:

$$T_{m.o.} = r_p.T_l = \frac{r_p d F_s}{2}\left(\mu \pm \frac{F_s X^2}{4EI}\right)\left(\frac{\mu}{\cos\theta} \pm \frac{l}{\pi d}\right) \tag{5.21}$$

4.2 THE CONTROLLER

Referring to previous work in the literature, different designs of tunable springs have been used and incorporated in the control of manipulators to modulate the stiffness of the end-point, while their positions are controlled independently (see for example [61]). In other word, the *position* control and *stiffness* of the actuation are decoupled by using a tunable spring in series with the conventional actuator of the joint. However, the novelty of this study is in the new application of tunable springs in order to decouple the *kinematics* of a fix-linkage mechanism such as the forceps (with the transmission ratio of motion r from its handle to the grasper) from its *kinetics* (determined by the force transmission ratio r' governed by the tunable spring and its controller) for the purpose of force control at the grasping point.

The objective of the controller is to supply the actuator with reference input X_{ref} as the *desired position* which is obtained from the required reference force F_{ref}, (Fig. 5.8), that in turn is defined to be the *desired force* F_{out} at the grasper which satisfies the two primary requirements of the system (i.e. defined as Req.I, and II in page 74), as:

$$F_{ref} \equiv F_{out} = \begin{cases} r'F_{in} & if: r'F_{in} \leq F_{lim} \\ F_{lim} & if: r'F_{in} > F_{lim} \end{cases} \tag{5.22}$$

Where r' is the desired force transmission (from the handle to the grasper), F_{lim} is the maximum limit of grasping force, and F_{ref} is the required grasping force (Fig. 5.8). In the control block diagram of (Fig. 5.8) and from the upper loop, F_{out}/F_{in} can be obtained as:

$$\frac{F_{out}}{F_{in}} = \frac{r}{1 + r^2 r_s^2 C_o K_s} \tag{5.23}$$

Assume the output of the lower loop (i.e. X) related to the actuator is tracking the desired value X_{ref} closely, so that it can be written that $X_{ref} \approx X$. Then by replacing $X = X_{ref}$ in Eq.(5.7) (i.e. $K_s = 24EI/X^3$) we can obtain X_{ref} as:

$$X_{ref} = \left(\frac{C}{\frac{rF_{in}}{F_{out}} - 1}\right)^{\frac{1}{3}} = \left(\frac{C}{\frac{rF_{in}}{F_{ref}} - 1}\right)^{\frac{1}{3}} \tag{5.24}$$

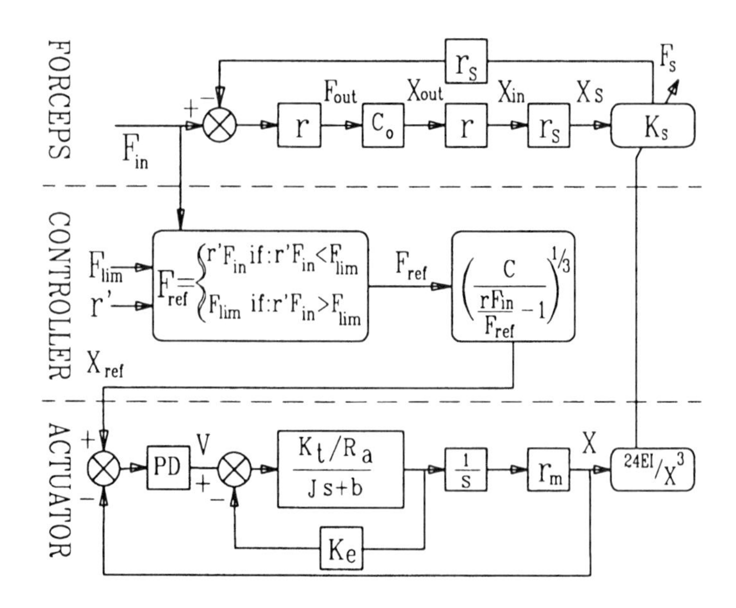

Figure 5.8. Block diagram of the integrated system.

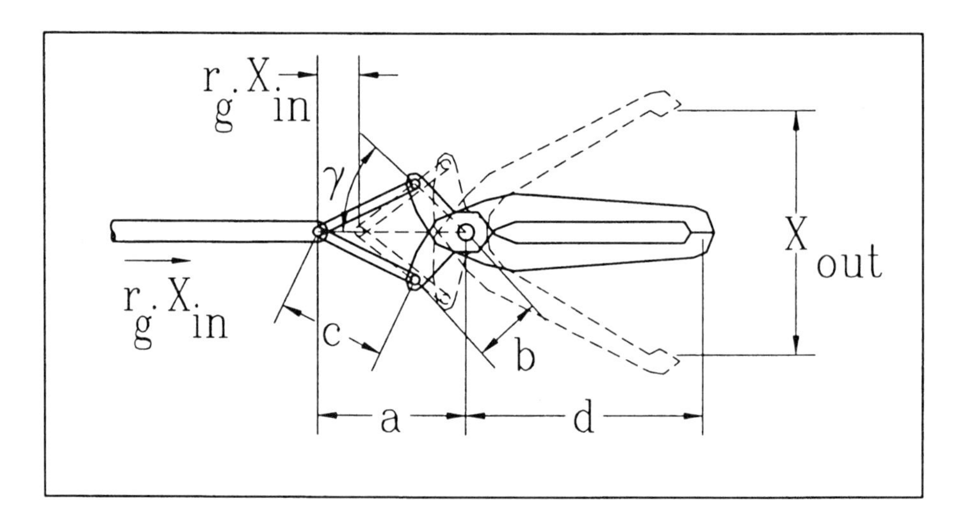

Figure 5.9. The mechanism and design parameters of the grasper.

Where $C = 24EIr^2r_s^2C_o$, and the compliance of environment $C_o = 1/K_o = X_{out}/F_{out}$. The compliance of environment C_o is assumed to be a constant, hence F_{out} and X_{out} have a linear relationship to each other.

In this book we assume the overall transmission of motion and force from handle to grasper to be linear, which means the transmission ratio $r = \frac{X_{in}}{X_{out}} = \frac{F_{out}}{F_{in}}$ is constant. The actual transmission based on the geom-

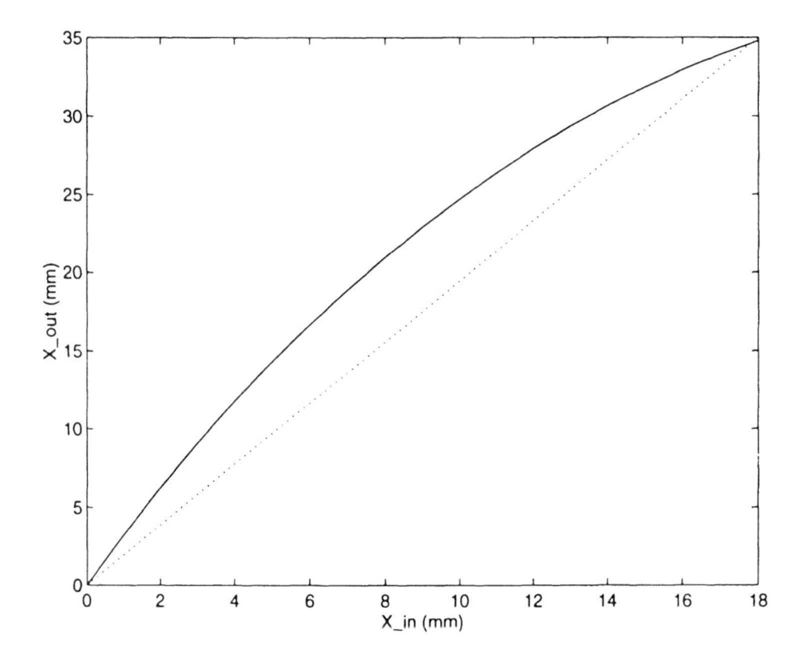

Figure 5.10. Displacement transmission from the handle to grasper.

etry of 4-bar linkage mechanism of grasper, Fig. 5.9 , can be formulated by:

$$c^2 = (a - r_g X_{in})^2 + b^2 - 2ab\cos\gamma, \text{ and } X_{out} = 2d\sin(\gamma_0 - \gamma)$$

Where a, b, c, d, and γ are geometrical parameters of the grasper (see Fig. 5.9), and r_g is the linear transmission ratio of motion from handle to the 4-bar linkage of the grasper. γ_0 is the initial value of γ when X_{in} is equal to zero in the above equations.

For typical design parameters of $a = 5, b = 4, c = 5, d = 32mm$, and $r_g = 0.19$(measured from the laparoscopic graspers of Ethicon, Johnson and Johnson), the transmission from handle X_{in} to grasper X_{out} based on the above equations is shown in Fig.5.10 (by the solid line) which can be approximated by linear functions (e.g. $X_{out} = X_{in}/r$, when $r = 0.51$ for the entire range of X_{in}, dotted line, Fig. 5.10).

5. SIMULATION RESULTS

For further study of the integrated system, it is numerically simulated using MATLAB - Simulink Toolbox (Fig. 5.11) based on the parameters given in Table.5.3 to verify its performance under simple linear ramp

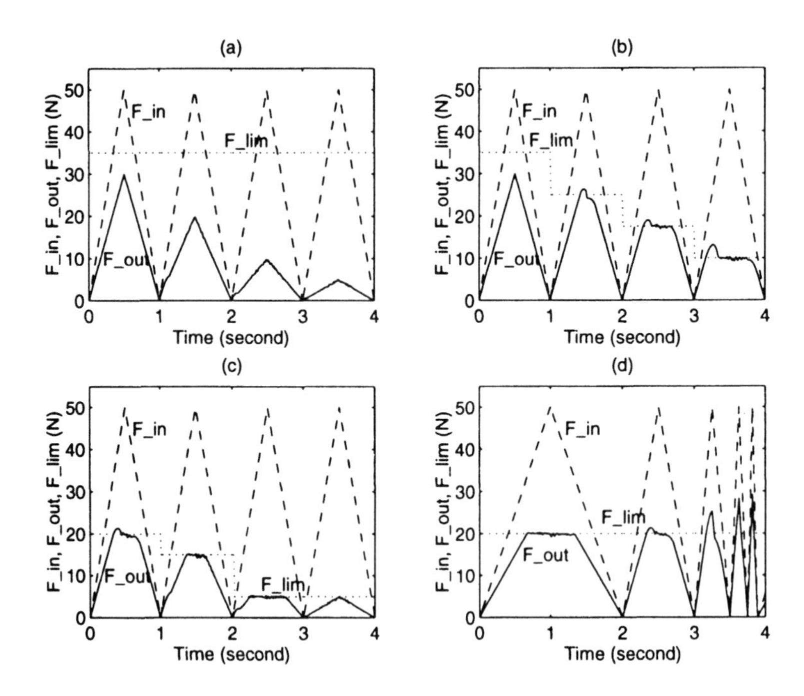

Figure 5.11. Simulation results of the integrated system.

loading. In Fig. 5.11(a) to (c), the linear variation of the handle force F_{in} from zero to maximum $50N$ as a ramp input has a frequency of 1Hz (dashed lines). The reduction effect of the force transmission ratio r' (with step values of 0.6, 0.4, 0.2, and 0.1 adjusted after each cycle) on the grasping force F_{out} (solid line) is shown in Fig. 5.11(a). In Fig. 5.11 (b), F_{lim} (dotted line) is decreased for each cycle, while in Fig. 5.11(c) both r', and F_{lim} are reduced to observe their combined effect on F_{out}. Finally in Fig. 5.11(d), the cycle period of input force is varied (i.e. 2, 1, 0.5, 0.25, and 0.12 sec.), while F_{lim} is kept constant to study the response of the system over the normal dynamic range of manipulation by the surgeon. The results of simulation (Fig.5.11a, b, and c) demonstrate the ability of the controller to observe both requirements of a) variability of force transmission from the handle to the grasper (Req.I), as well as, b) adjustability of the maximum force at the grasper (Req.II), simultaneously. The simulation results are further discussed in conjunction with the bandwidth analysis (Sec. 6), and also with the experimental results (Sec. 7).

Table 5.3. Simulation parameters of the haptic grasper.

Grasper	r	Transmission ratio from handle to grasper	-	0.7
	X_{in}^{max}	Maximum actuation of handle	mm	14.
	X_{out}^{max}	Maximum movement of Grasper	mm	20.
	r_s	Transmission ratio from handle to spring	-	0.05
Spring	X_s^{max}	Maximum deflection of spring	mm	0.7
	L	Total length of leaf spring	mm	125.
	w	Width of leaf spring	mm	12.7
	t	Thickness of leaf spring	mm	1.6
	E	Module of elasticity	GPa	127.
Actuation mechanism	X^{max}	Total actuation stroke	mm	80.
	d	Diameter of lead screw	mm	6.
	l	Pitch of lead screw	mm	1.
	r_p	Pulleys transmission ratio	-	2
	r_m	total transmission ratio ($l.r_p/2\pi$) from motor to lead screw	mm/rad.	0.32
Motor	K_t	Torque constant	N.m/A	0.05
	K_e	Electric constant	V.sec/rad	0.05
	J	Rotor moment of inertia	$N.m.sec.^2$	$2. \times 10^{-6}$
	b	Damping constant	$N.m.sec.$	1.4×10^{-4}
	R_a	Resistance of armature	Ω	1.2
PD Gains	K_p	Proportional Gain	V/mm	8.
	K_d	Differential Gain	$V/mm.sec.$	3.
Environment	C_0	Compliance	mm/N	0.65

6. BANDWIDTH ANALYSIS

The results of simulation (Fig. 5.11) confirm that the tunable spring design has the potential to meet both of the requirements for quasi-static manipulation[5] of the tissue, as well as more dynamic manipulations up to 2 Hz bandwidth. However, above 2 Hz (Fig. 5.11d) the force limit F_{lim} related to Req.II starts to deteriorate.

On the other hand, the system continues to observe Req.I (as the transmission ratio r' is varied) independent of the dynamics of input force F_{in}. This can be shown by substituting $F_{ref} = r'F_{in}$ (5.22) in Eq.5.24 which simplifies to:

[5]When the variation of manipulating force over time is very gradual near zero(e.g. $\leq 0.2Hz$ for the tissue manipulation).

$$X_{ref} = \left(\frac{C}{\frac{rF_{in}}{F_{ref}} - 1}\right)^{\frac{1}{3}} = \left(\frac{C}{\frac{rF_{in}}{r'F_{in}} - 1}\right)^{\frac{1}{3}} = \left(\frac{C}{\frac{r}{r'} - 1}\right)^{\frac{1}{3}}$$

Which is independent of F_{in}, and this means for every occasional manual adjustment of r' by the surgeon, there is a single adjustment of X_{ref} to meet Req.I independent of F_{in} and its bandwidth.

To determine analytically the operating frequency range of the system, analysis related to Req.II (when the force limit F_{lim} being exceeded) is performed.

In this regard, multiply both sides of Eq.5.23 by F_{in}/F_{ref} to obtain:

$$\frac{F_{out}}{F_{ref}} = \frac{r.F_{in}/F_{ref}}{1 + r^2 r_s^2 C_o K_s} = \frac{f}{1 + r^2 r_s^2 C_o K_s} \tag{5.25}$$

Where $f \equiv r.F_{in}/F_{ref}$, and since we are considering the bandwidth under the condition of Req.II, we have $F_{ref} = F_{lim}$ (5.22). By substituting for F_{ref} we can then obtain $f = r.F_{in}/F_{lim}$.

On the other hand, K_s based on Eq. (5.7) can be linearized as:

$$K_s^{(X)} \approx K_s^{(X_{ref})} + K_s^{'(X_{ref})}(X - X_{ref}) = \frac{24EI}{X_{ref}^3}(4 - 3\frac{X}{X_{ref}}) \tag{5.26}$$

Also, the transfer function of $\frac{X}{X_{ref}}$ based on the outer actuator loop (Fig. 5.8) is:

$$\frac{X}{X_{ref}} = \frac{1}{As^2 + Bs + 1} \tag{5.27}$$

Where $A = JR_a/K_t Pr_m$, and $B = K_e/Pr_m$. After substituting Eq.5.26, and 5.27, in 5.25 we obtain:

$$\frac{F_{out}}{F_{ref}} = K_G \frac{As^2 + Bs + 1}{As^2 + Bs + K_G} \tag{5.28}$$

Where $K_G = f/(4f - 3)$.

The Bode diagrams of Eq.5.28, and its roots locus for changing f, are shown in Fig. 5.12. It is evident from Fig. 5.12a, and 5.12b that the output force tracks the reference value F_{lim} with very small deviation (less than 10%) and phase difference (less than 10°) in the range of 0-2Hz bandwidth. However, the deviation and phase difference grows quite fast above 3Hz, which is the functional bandwidth limit of the system.

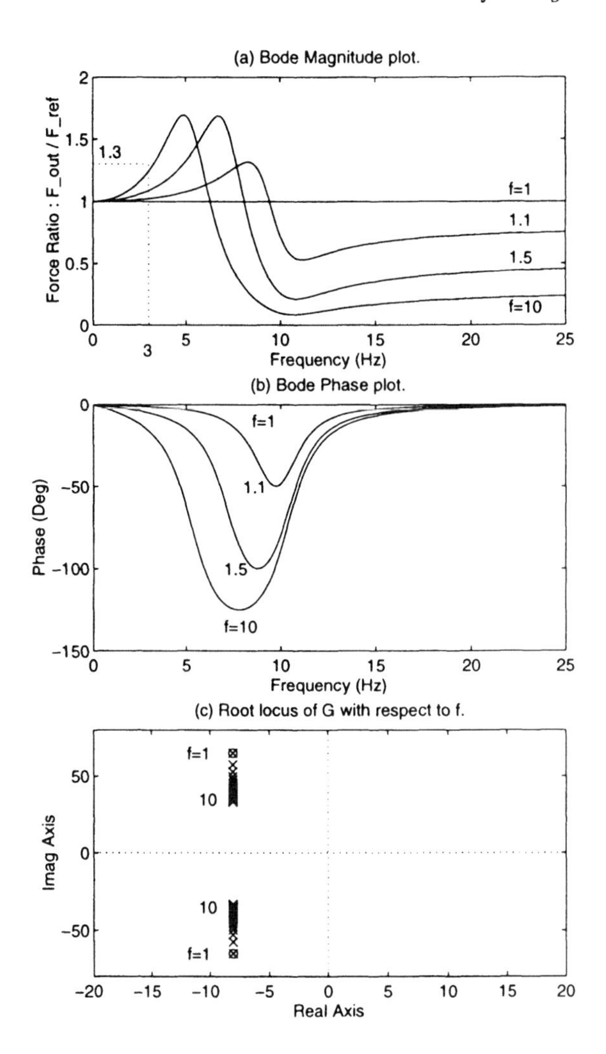

Figure 5.12. Dynamic response of the system.

7. EXPERIMENTAL RESULTS

The above analysis and simulation results demonstrate the potential for the application of tunable springs in a design of a haptic interface, which meets the preset goals and requirements adequately. This has convinced us to build a prototype for experimental study and proof of concept.

The experimental set-up consists of a laparoscopic grasper, mounted on a base plate, whose modified handle is coupled with the tunable spring (Fig. 5.13). The design parameters of the grasper, and the tunable spring are given in Table 5.4.

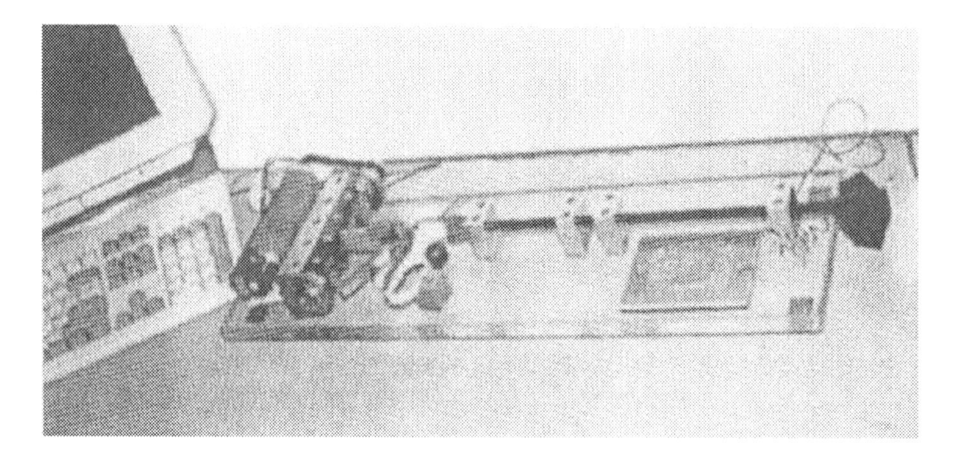

Figure 5.13. The experimental set up of the haptic grasper for laparoscopy.

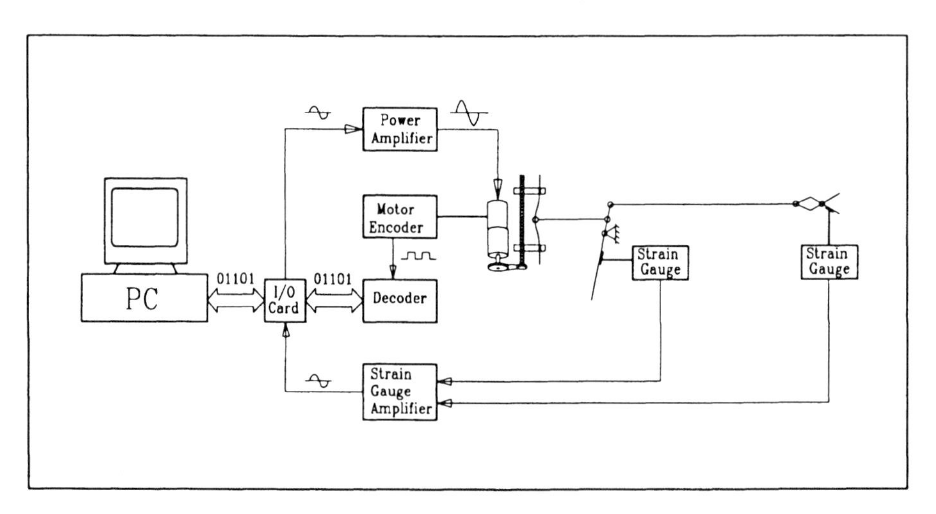

Figure 5.14. Schematic block diagram of the tunable spring, grasper, and electronic hardware.

The actuator of the tunable spring is a DC motor, driven by a pulse width modulation (PWM) servo amplifier, which is interfaced through a PC with an I/O card (Table.5.5). For force measurements, two semiconductor strain gauges are mounted at the handle and grasper, and their signals after conditioning (10 Hz low pass cut off filter) are the input of the computer through the I/O card (Table.5.5). The schematic block diagram of the experimental set-up is shown in Fig. 5.14, and further information for different components of the system is provided in Table.5.5.

Table 5.4. Design parameters of the experimental prototype.

Grasper	r	Transmission ratio from handle to grasper	-	0.58
	X_{in}^{max}	Maximum actuation of handle	mm	13.
	X_{out}^{max}	Maximum movement of Grasper	mm	22.5
	r_s	Transmission ratio from handle to spring	-	0.046
Spring	X_s^{max}	Maximum deflection of spring	mm	0.75
	L	Total length of leaf spring	mm	140.
	w	Width of leaf spring	mm	12.7
	t	Thickness of leaf spring	mm	1.6
	E	Module of elasticity	GPa	127.
Actuation mechanism	X^{max}	Total actuation stroke	mm	84.
	d	Diameter of lead screw	mm	6.
	l	Pitch of lead screw	mm	1.
	r_p	Pulleys transmission ratio	-	2
	r_m	total transmission ratio from motor to lead screw	mm/rad	0.32
Motor	K_t	Torque constant	N.m/A	0.105
	K_e	Electric constant	V.sec/rad	0.11
	J	Rotor moment of inertia	$N.m.sec.^2$	4.2×10^{-6}
	b	Damping constant	$N.m.sec.$	2.8×10^{-4}
	R_a	Resistance of armature	Ω	1.9
Environment	C_0	Compliance (polyurethane)	mm/N	0.75

A set of experimental tests have been designed to demonstrate the ability of the system to meet our two primary requirements (Req.I and II), as well as to establish the bandwidth range of the system as follows:

Experiment 1 - To demonstrate that Req.I is satisfied, the experimental procedure is to apply force pulses to the handle of grasper while setting different levels of the transmission ratio r' (similar to the simulation, Fig. 5.11a). To meet Req.I, The transmitted force F_{out} at the grasper must be proportional to F_{in} based on the desired transmission ratio r'.

Experiment 2 - The ability of the haptic interface to meet Req.II is verified by setting the limit of grasping force (F_{lim}) at different levels while exerting same pulsating forces at the handle (F_{in}) for each of the settings (similar to the simulation, Fig. 5.11b). To meet Req.II,

Table 5.5. Electronic hardware and software of the experimental set-up.

Motor Encoder	Type:	optical encoder, quadrature signal, TTL
	Input:	5 VDC
	Output:	512 pulses/revolution
Motor Drive	Type:	Pulse width modulation (PWM) servo amplifier
	Peak output:	+/- 80 Volts 25 Amp.
	Continuous output:	Max. 12.5 Amp.
	Input:	+/- 15 Volts
	Gain:	2.8 Amp./Volt
I/O card	Type:	8 Bits digital I/O interface, TTL
	Inputs:	6 Channels for A/D
	Outputs:	2 Channels for D/A
	Bandwidth:	Max. 4KHz/channel
Strain Gauge	Type:	Semi-conductor
	Gauge factor:	130.
	Resistance:	120. Ω
	S.G. Drive:	Constant current (10 mA)
	Amp. Gain:	15
	Output:	18.5 mV/N for grasper strain gauge
	Input:	15.0 mV/N for handle strain gauge
Hardware	PC computer:	Pentium 100MHz, 16 Mb RAM
Software Drive	Filtering:	Strain gauge 10 Hz low pass cut off filter
	PD Controller:	Proportional gain $K_P = 5V/mm$
		Differential gain $K_d = 2V/mm.Sec.$

the grasping force F_{out} must not exceed the desired limit F_{lim}, and the spring must absorb any additional force applied at the handle.

Experiment 3 - The bandwidth of the system can be tested experimentally by applying input pulses at the handle with gradual increase in its bandwidth frequency (similar to the simulation, Fig. 5.11d). The operating bandwidth range of the system can be established experimentally as the input frequency of pulses at the handle increases while the grasping force F_{out} can be limited based on F_{lim} setting.

Initial results of Exp.1 were not able to show that Req.I is met (Fig. 5.15). In this experiment, although r' was varied from 0.2 to 0.5 (Fig. 5.15a), and the controller was actuating correctly based on the desired X_{ref}

(Fig. 5.15b), the actual transmission ratio[6] r_{act} did not have any correlation with the desired levels of r' (Fig. 5.15c). In fact F_{out} remained almost unaffected and stayed at the same level independent of r' variation (Fig. 5.15a). This was caused mainly due to the backlash and free clearances in the joints of mechanical linkages. In fact, the total deflection of tunable spring by the movement of handle is about 0.7mm (due to low transmission of $r_s = 0.045$), and any minute amount of clearance and free play in the connecting linkage of the spring and the grasper, as well as any clearance in the supporting slides of spring would prevent the transfer of the required force from the spring to the grasper. Furthermore this can be explained in Fig. 5.15c, by more detailed examination of r_{act} plots. In all four pulsing cycles of r_{act} shown in Fig. 5.15c, initially the transmission ratio r_{act} reaches its first peak of about 0.57 (i.e. equal to r, the fixed mechanical transmission ratio from the handle to grasper), which indicates that due to the free play at the start, the grasper is acting as a stand alone mechanism receiving no effect from the tunable spring. Then gradually r_{act} drops when the free play is eventually absorbed by the movement of handle. However due to the partial loss of actuation, the value of r_{act} can not reach the low desired settings (e.g. 0.2 and 0.3 Fig. 5.15c). Furthermore, the cause of the second high peak of r_{act} is due to friction in the mechanism when the handle is being released (Fig. 5.15a), and the manipulating forces F_{in} is dropping to relatively low levels. This means when F_{in} has low values, F_{out} still remains at its relatively higher values due to friction, which causes $r_{act} = F_{out}/F_{in}$ to increase sharply to above 1.5 .

The second problem causing the mechanism not to behave according to the desired requirements was the deformation of the base plate under high forces between the actuated spring and the handle (observed in Exp.2, Fig.5.16). The baseplate (where the grasper and tunable spring are mounted), was initially made of Plexiglas material, which bent under the load, causing the upper bound of stiffness of the tunable spring to be limited to the relatively low stiffness of the baseplate.

The combination of the problem of low stiffness of the base plate, and the problem of clearances in the joints, prevented sufficient amount of force F_s to be developed by the spring in Exp.2. Consequently, the force limit F_{lim} could not be observed by F_{out} as required Fig. 5.16a (while the actuation of spring X follows closely the desired actuation X_{ref}, Fig. 5.16b).

[6] The actual transmission ratio is defined as: $r_{act} = F_{out}/F_{in}$ where F_{out}, and F_{in} are the actual measured forces at the grasper and the handle respectively.

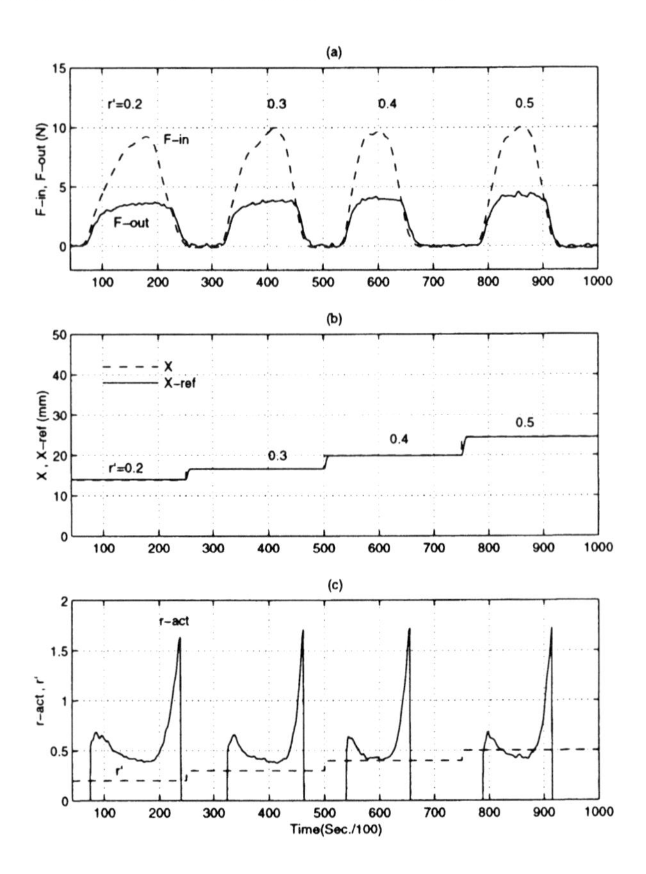

Figure 5.15. Changing of r' with no effect on the grasping force F_{out}.

In order to address both problems, the design of prototype was revised by a)changing the base plate from Plexiglas to aluminum, thus increasing its stiffness by a factor of 5, b) pre-loading the linkage that links the handle to the tunable spiring, in order to eliminate clearances of joints and free plays.

The design modifications proved to be effective and provided satisfactory experimental results. Exp.1 was performed again with results shown in Fig. 5.17, where F_{out} decreases proportionally as the setting r' is decreased from 0.4 to 0.1 (Fig. 5.17a). The average of actual transmission ratio $r_{act} = F_{out}/F_{in}$ in Fig. 5.17b corresponds to the desired setting r'. In this plot (Fig. 5.17b), there are two peaks at the start and end of each r_{act} cycle. The second peaks are caused by the friction when the handle is released (as described above for Fig. 5.15c). However, the first set of peaks is caused by the friction due to the pre-loading (as the trade off for backlash elimination). It must be noted that the dotted portions of r_{act} in Fig. 5.17c (e.g. from t=2.4 to 3. sec., as well as at

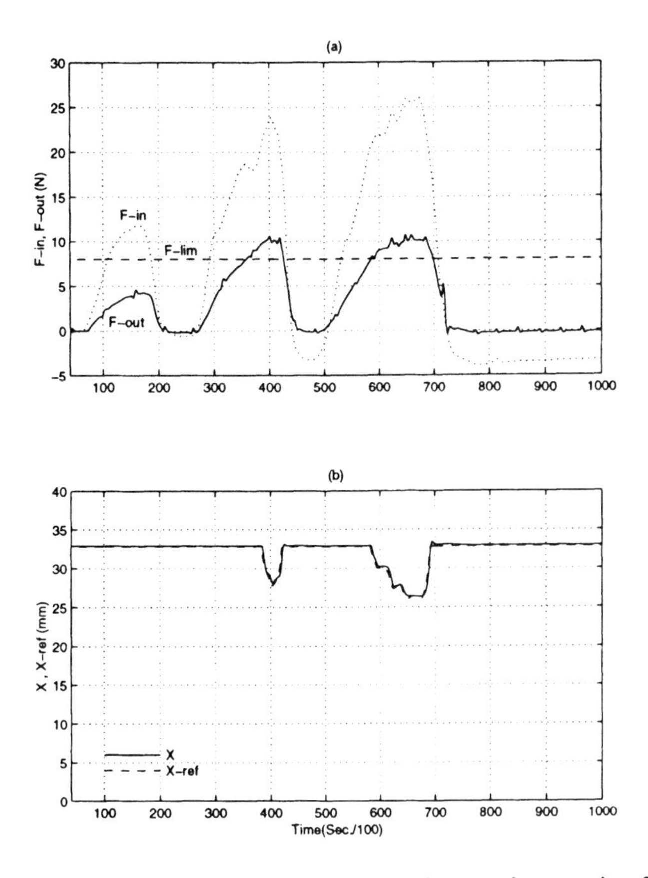

Figure 5.16. Force setting F_{lim} with no limiting effect on the grasping force F_{out}.

t=5. and 7.6 sec.) correspond to very low levels of force in the linkages when the friction force as noise is dominant, and do not have any operational significant.

The experimental results of Exp.2, after modifications, agree with the design goal of limiting the grasping force F_{out} based on the desired limit of F_{lim} (Fig. 5.18) at different levels. This is obtained by the actuation of the tunable spring (Fig. 5.18b) as soon as F_{out} reaches F_{lim} as described earlier, so that the spring absorbs any additional force applied at the handle.

The third set of experimental results of Exp.3 demonstrate that the goal of limiting grasping force F_{out} is achieved up to the bandwidth of 2Hz (the first three peaks, Fig. 5.19a). Above 2Hz, the system can not limit F_{out} fully, since the actuation of tunable spring X can not track the desired actuation X_{ref} (e.g. the last 6 pulses, Fig. 5.19b). Although the partial actuation at the higher frequency ($> 2Hz$, Fig. 5.19a) can

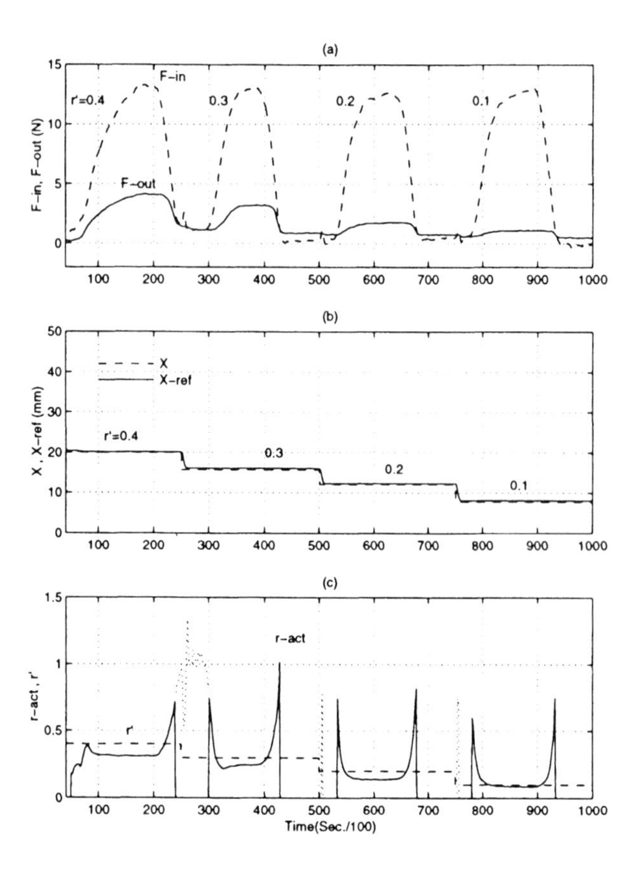

Figure 5.17. The changing effect of r' on the grasping force F_{out}.

not totally limit the output force F_{out}, it reduces the transmission ratio significantly so that it prevents a substantial increase of F_{out} above the limit F_{lim} (e.g. 3 to 5 Hz pulses, Fig. 5.19a).

The experimental results fully confirm the simulation and analytical results that are discussed in the next section.

8. DISCUSSION AND FURTHER DEVELOPMENTS

The results of analysis(Eq.5.28) and simulation (Fig.5.11) show that the tunable spring design has the potential to meet both of the requirements (Page. 74) from quasi-static manipulations of tissue to more dynamic manipulations up to 1-2 Hz bandwidth. Above 2 Hz (Fig.5.11d), the force limit F_{lim} (i.e. Req.II) starts to deteriorate.

The experimental results(Fig.5.17 to 19) fully confirm the simulation and analytical results both in terms of the adjustable proportional trans-

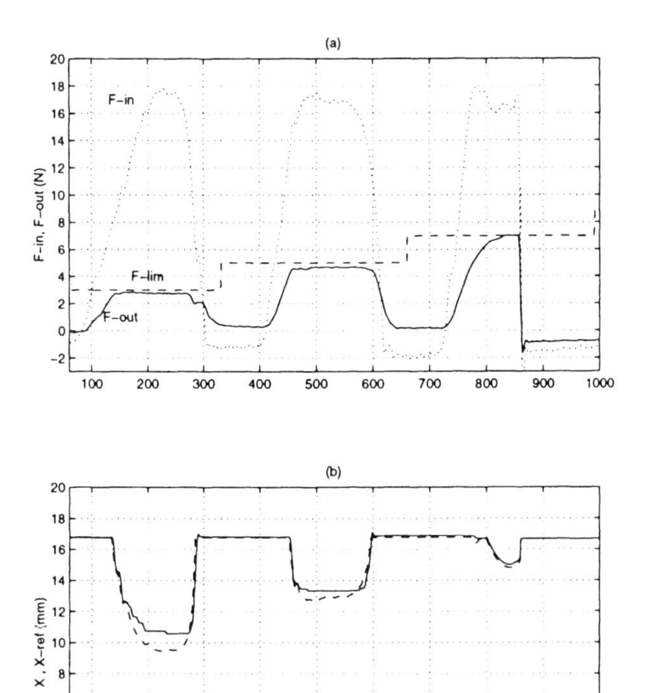

Figure 5.18. The effect of force limit F_{lim} on the output force F_{out}.

mission (Req.I) and the adjustable maximum limit for F_{out} (Req.II) as well as the operating bandwidth range of the tunable spring. However, the operation of the system can be enhanced by adding position sensors to obtain the displacement of the grasper. This position sensing would enable us to compute the stiffness of the environment in real time by dividing the measured grasping force by the displacement. The measurements provide an accurate estimation of stiffness, rather than the initial assumption of constant environmental stiffness, which in turn helps the controller to perform even better and meet the two requirements more closely.

In general, for high fidelity of force reflection to human hands, the system should have adequate bandwidth ($> 50Hz$), in order to reflect high frequency "jitter" or vibration when interacting with "hard" objects or rigid environment[48]. Tunable springs inherently do not have high bandwidth due to properties of the mechanical actuation of the spring

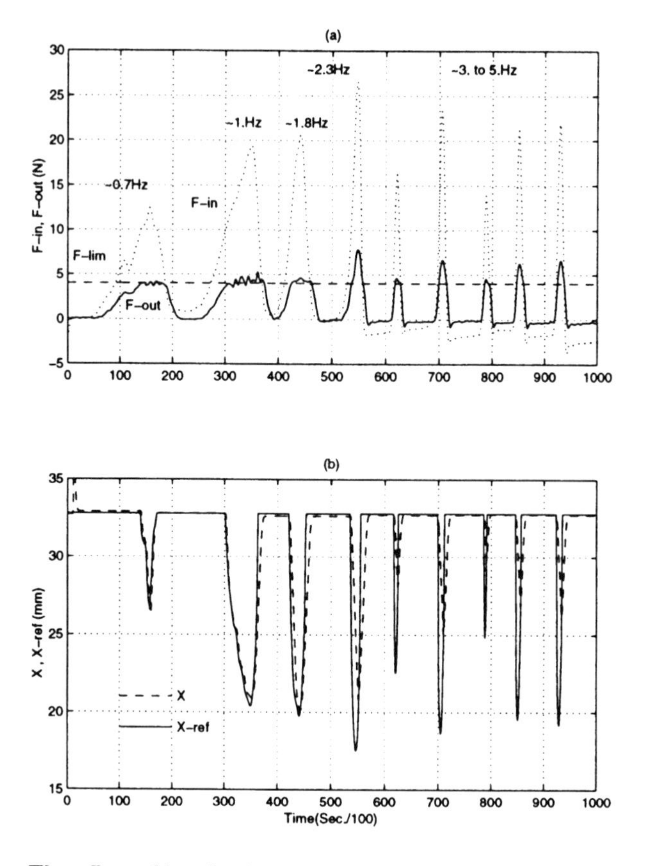

Figure 5.19. The effect of bandwidth on the grasping force with limit F_{lim}.

(such as the travel time required for the spring to respond, inertia, and backlash). However, in this application for endoscopic graspers, the interacting environment (i.e. tissue, not considering the needle as the only hard object to be manipulated in the suturing task) is soft, and does not require a relatively high bandwidth. Thus the bandwidth in this application is much lower (in the order of 2-3 Hz) limited to the frequency of the hand movements of the surgeon to manipulate the tissue.

The tunable spring design can have applications in other force reflection master-slave systems, either as *passive mechanical* systems (similar to laparoscopic graspers), or *actuated tele-operated* systems with low bandwidth requirements. As an improvement, the higher bandwidth forces/displacements sensed at the slave site from the environment (such as minute vibrations caused by the collision of slave with rigid objects) can be reflected to the hand of operator separately by using piezo-electric actuators[90] at the handle of the master-arm. This is a complementary synthesis of tunable-springs (to reflect high amplitude force/displacement with low bandwidth), and piezo-electric actuators (to reflect low amplitude force/displacement with high bandwidth) to provide a wider and better haptic interface with the hand of the operator.

Chapter 6

ROBOTIC EXTENDERS

Remote manipulation in laparoscopy introduces constraints on the dexterity of the hand motion due to: a) spherical movements of tool at the port of entry on the abdomen (Ch.2), and b) lack of dexterity inside the abdomen (Ch.3). Chapter 2 and 3 presented some design concepts which can be used individually, while offering the surgeon added dexterity. However, by extending the designs into the field of *robotics*, it is possible to provide the bases for more advanced developments in laparoscopic systems.

There are a number of works in the literature which address robotic applications for laparoscopy. These applications can be categorized in two main types of robotic extenders:

I) Automated Positioners: This type is basically a positioner for laparoscopic tools and a navigating system. In addition to locking tools in a desired configuration, it also can reposition the tool to a previously stored location (e.g. for changing the angle of endoscopic view to a previously stored orientation). This type of positioner is also commercially available from Computer Motion Inc. (AESOP units, Fig.6.1)[14].

Taylor *et al*, at IBM Thomas J. Watson Research center [86] have developed an automated positioner with a parallelogram configuration to provide remote centre of rotation at the incision point. Also the commercial development (EndoSista) by Armstrong Projects, England[34] is a specially designed positioner to control laparoscopic view directly by head movements of the surgeon.

II) Tele-Operated Extenders: One of the main areas of potential application for robotic extenders in laparoscopy, is the field of tele-

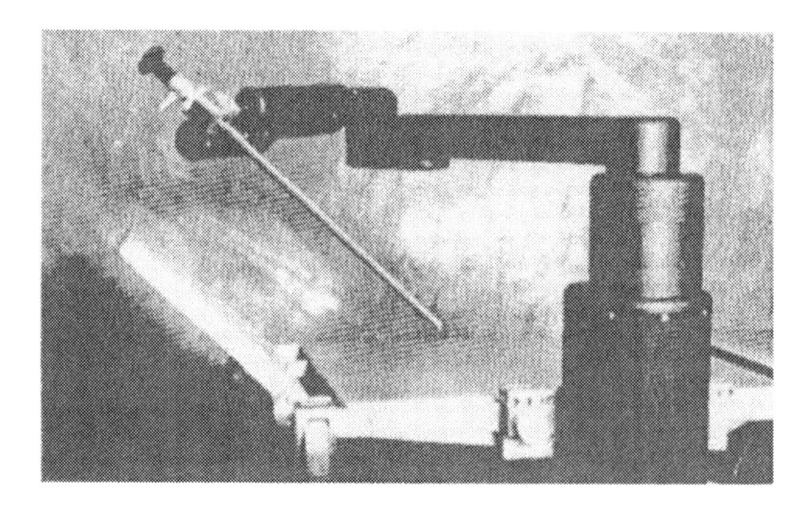

Figure 6.1. Robotic positioner AESOP for laparoscopy, by Computer Motion Inc.

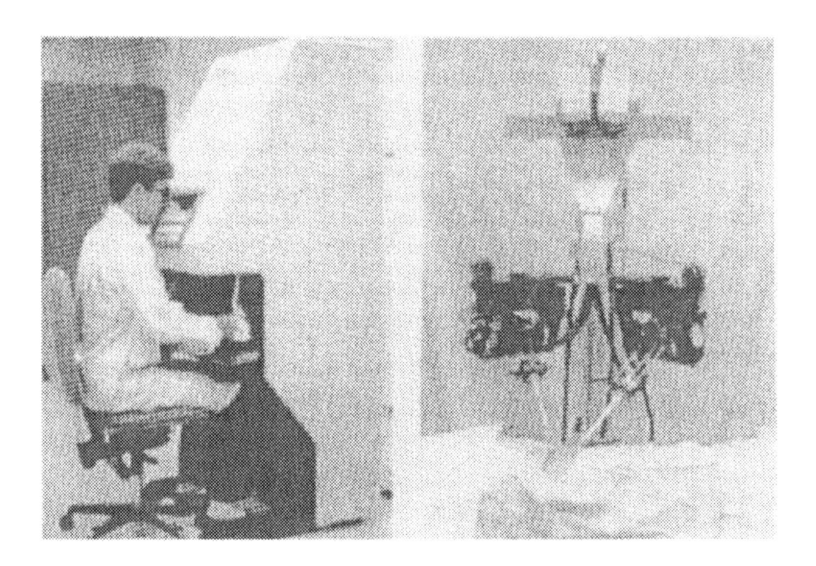

Figure 6.2. Robotic tele-surgical system by SRI International.

operated master-slave system. As it was stated, laparoscopic surgery with the associated inverse hand motion and limited force sensing is very unnatural to perform and physically demanding. This can motivate the design and development of tele-operated extenders so that the surgeon can control the direct motion of the tool's tip on the monitor, instead of reverse motion at the handle. The master-slave robotic system controls the movements of the slave extender inside the abdominal cavity by hand movements of the surgeon through a master arm on a tele-surgical workstation[32].

There are also other research works proposing the general concept of tele-surgical workstations for laparoscopy, which are based on master-slave tele-operated systems[58][64]. However, there has not been any specific design for implementation or experimental developments for laparoscopy. The only experimental tele-operated surgical development belongs to SRI International[39]. However their current design configuration is only suitable for open surgery (Fig.6.2), since it does not have any DOF to perform spherical movements at the port of entry which is a primary requirement for laparoscopy[1].

In this chapter, our main effort is to study laparoscopic robotic extenders, and specify their requirements for any of the above applications. This includes the kinematic study, as well as planned constrained motion of such extenders, in order to provide the basis for future robotic developments.

1. CONFIGURATION OF ROBOTIC EXTENDERS

The design configuration of robotic extenders for laparoscopic applications (e.g. Type I, or II, mentioned above) should generally meet the two primary requirements:

1. To comply with the kinematic constraint at the port of entry.
2. To provide sufficient DOF inside the abdomen for the specific surgical task.

The *first requirement* is also related to the type synthesis similar to the one carried out in Ch.2. Those results can be used here, and the same mechanism of concentric spherical mechanism can also provide the remote centre of rotation for the robotic extender. The only difference here would be the addition of actuators to the previously passive joints.

Compared to the above mechanical solution, there is another robotic solution for creating a remote centre of rotation at the port of entry. This approach is based on controlled simultaneous motion of two or more joints of the robotic arm, so that the contact point of the extender at the incision point on abdomen remains stationary while having its 4 DOF at

[1]At the time of completion of this book, other telesurgical prototypes have been developed in various research centers.For example see: (http://www.intuitivesurgical.com.) and (http://robotics.eecs.berkeley.edu/mcenk/medical/).

the port of entry. This is how AESOP[14] functions, and kinematically simulates a pseudo-spherical joint as a remote center of rotation at the abdomen. However, this approach has some disadvantage as follows: *In the case of any failure in one of the simultaneously controlled axes (due to some motion limit of joints, singularity, or software/hardware failure in one of the drive units), the incision point at the port of entry could be damaged. Also, the actuation drive computer requires additional computing power to drive all the joints simultaneously in real time, which means more expensive control and computer systems.*

Hence in this study, only the type of laparoscopic robotic extenders with the mechanical concentric spherical mechanism is considered for the purpose of creating remote center of rotation at the port of entry.

The *second requirement* of providing sufficient DOF inside the abdomen, is related to the type and functionality of the extender. The following additional DOF and joints configurations are required in the case of the two types of robotic extenders described in this study (i.e. Type I, and II), in order for them to function:

Case I - Required DOF for Automated Positioners

Generally laparoscopic positioners are used either for positioning the laparoscope, or surgical tools (such as retractors, graspers, etc), which both cases require two positioning DOF (i.e. θ_1, and θ_2, Fig.6.3). In the case of the laparoscope, 2 additional DOF at the port of entry are needed. One DOF for the rotational adjustment of laparoscope around its longitudinal axis (θ_3), so that the image on the monitor obtains an upright orientation. The second DOF for translating the laparoscope in and out of abdomen for zooming purposes. Also, in the case of surgical tools, the same 2 DOF are required for proper orientation and axial reach at the surgical site. Therefore for this type of positioner, generally a total of 4 DOF (i.e. $\theta_1, \theta_2, \theta_3$, and l at the port of entry, Fig.6.3) is adequate. The design of extender can be implemented by adding the 2 actuated joints (i.e. C, and D) to the distal end of concentric spherical mechanism (from Ch.2) with actuated joints A and B as shown schematically in Fig.6.3.

Case II - Required DOF for Tele-Operated Extenders

The current laparoscopic tools with rigid stem have only 4 DOF (Ch.3) and a tele-operated slave extender with rigid stem would also have 4 DOF similar to Case I (i.e. 3 DOF, θ_1, θ_2, l for positioning, and 1 DOF, θ_3, for orientation). However, by incorporating flexible stem (synthesized in Ch.3) as an added end-effector to the end of the extender (Fig.6.4), it is possible to have all 6 DOF (i.e. with

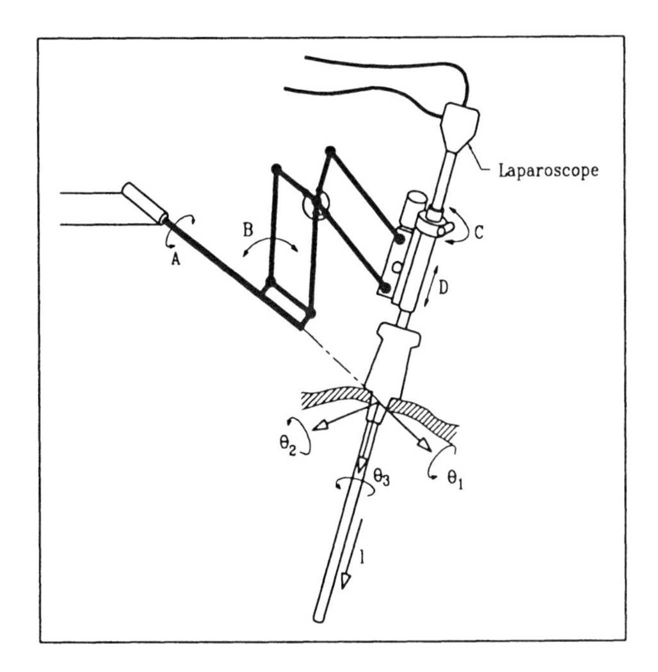

Figure 6.3. Schematic of the robotic extender with 4 DOF.

the two additional DOF for orientation, θ_4 and θ_5) to manipulate the surgical tissues without any kinematic constraint. This would be a complementary step compared to the design of Case I (Fig.6.3). It is obtained by combining the concentric spherical mechanism (Ch.2), and the flexible stem designs (Ch.3). Joints A, B, C, and D function identically to Case I, while E provides actuation for the joint on stem (i.e. θ_4). A flexible shaft can transmit both of the actuations F and G, for rotation (i.e. θ_5), and grasping action respectively (Fig.6.4).

In the following section, the kinematics of the above combined design configuration is further studied, which includes homogeneous coordinates transformation, forward and inverse kinematics, singularity study, and constraint motion of such robotic extenders.

2. KINEMATICS OF THE EXTENDER

The kinematic aspects of the above laparoscopic extender (Case II) with 6 DOF is studied here, and Case I with 4 DOF can be considered as a special case of Case II (when $\theta_4 = \theta_5 = 0$). In this study, the coordinate transformations from the base (i.e. point B, Fig 6.6) to the distal end of extender (point E) are considered. A commonly used convention for selecting frames of reference in robotic applications is through

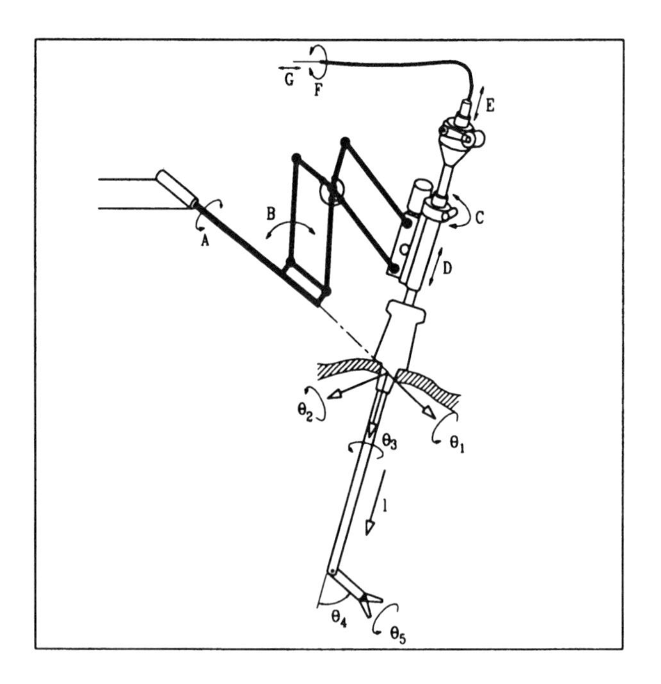

Figure 6.4. Schematic of the robotic extender with 6 DOF.

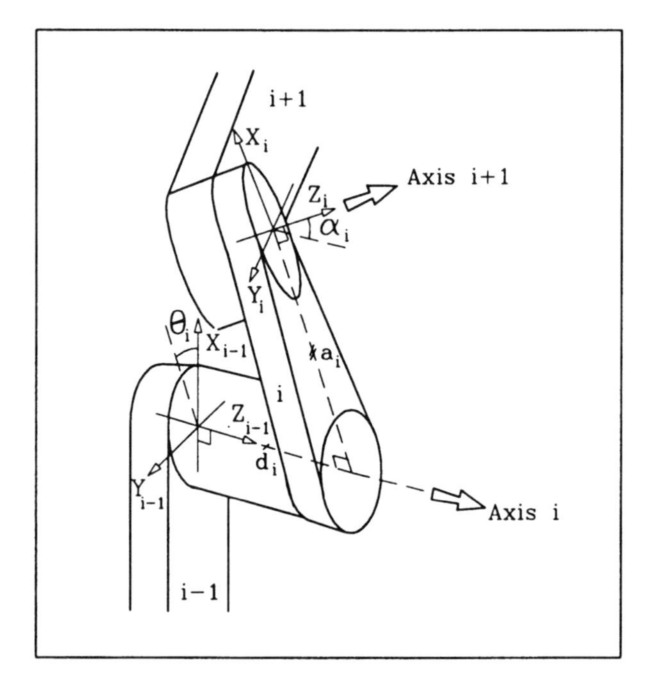

Figure 6.5. The parameters of i-th link of a manipulator based on Denavit-Hartenberg convention.

Table 6.1. The parameters of laparoscopic extender.

Link/Joint	a_i	α_i	d_i	θ_i
1	0	$-90°$	0	θ_1
2	0	$90°$	0	$\theta_2 - 90°$
3	0	0	0	θ_3
4	0	$-90°$	l	0
5	0	$90°$	0	θ_4
6	0	0	l_e	θ_5

the Denavit-Hartenberg (or D-H) convention[4][78]. Based on the convention, various parameters of link i are defined as: θ_i the joint angle between X-axes of frame i and i-1 (Fig.6.5); α_i, the twist angle between joints axes i and i+1; a_i, the length of common normal of joints axes i and i+1 as the length of the link; and d_i, the offset along axis i from the origin of frame i-1 to the base of the common normal[94] (Fig.6.5). The parameters of the laparoscopic extender (Fig.6.6) a_i, α_i, d_i, and θ_i (for i=1,6) are given in Table 6.1. The homogeneous transformation $\mathbf{A}_i$ along each link is defined as:

$$\mathbf{A}_i = Rot_{z,\theta_i} Trans_{z,d_i} Trans_{x,a_i} Rot_{x,\alpha_i}$$

Or,

$$\mathbf{A}_i = \begin{bmatrix} C\theta_i & -S\theta_i C\alpha_i & S\theta_i S\alpha_i & a_i C\theta_i \\ S\theta_i & C\theta_i C\alpha_i & -C\theta_i S\alpha_i & a_i S\theta_i \\ 0 & S\alpha_i & C\alpha_i & d_i \\ 0 & 0 & 0 & 1 \end{bmatrix}$$

By substituting the parameters for each joint from Table 6.1, we can obtain the following transformation matrices:

$$\mathbf{A}_1 = \begin{bmatrix} C_1 & 0 & -S_1 & 0 \\ S_1 & 0 & C_1 & 0 \\ 0 & -1 & 0 & 0 \\ 0 & 0 & 0 & 1 \end{bmatrix} \qquad \mathbf{A}_2 = \begin{bmatrix} S_2 & 0 & -C_2 & 0 \\ -C_2 & 0 & -S_2 & 0 \\ 0 & 1 & 0 & 0 \\ 0 & 0 & 0 & 1 \end{bmatrix}$$

$$\mathbf{A}_3 = \begin{bmatrix} C_3 & -S_3 & 0 & 0 \\ S_3 & C_3 & 0 & 0 \\ 0 & 0 & 1 & 0 \\ 0 & 0 & 0 & 1 \end{bmatrix} \qquad \mathbf{A}_4 = \begin{bmatrix} 1 & 0 & 0 & 0 \\ 0 & 0 & 1 & 0 \\ 0 & -1 & 0 & l \\ 0 & 0 & 0 & 1 \end{bmatrix}$$

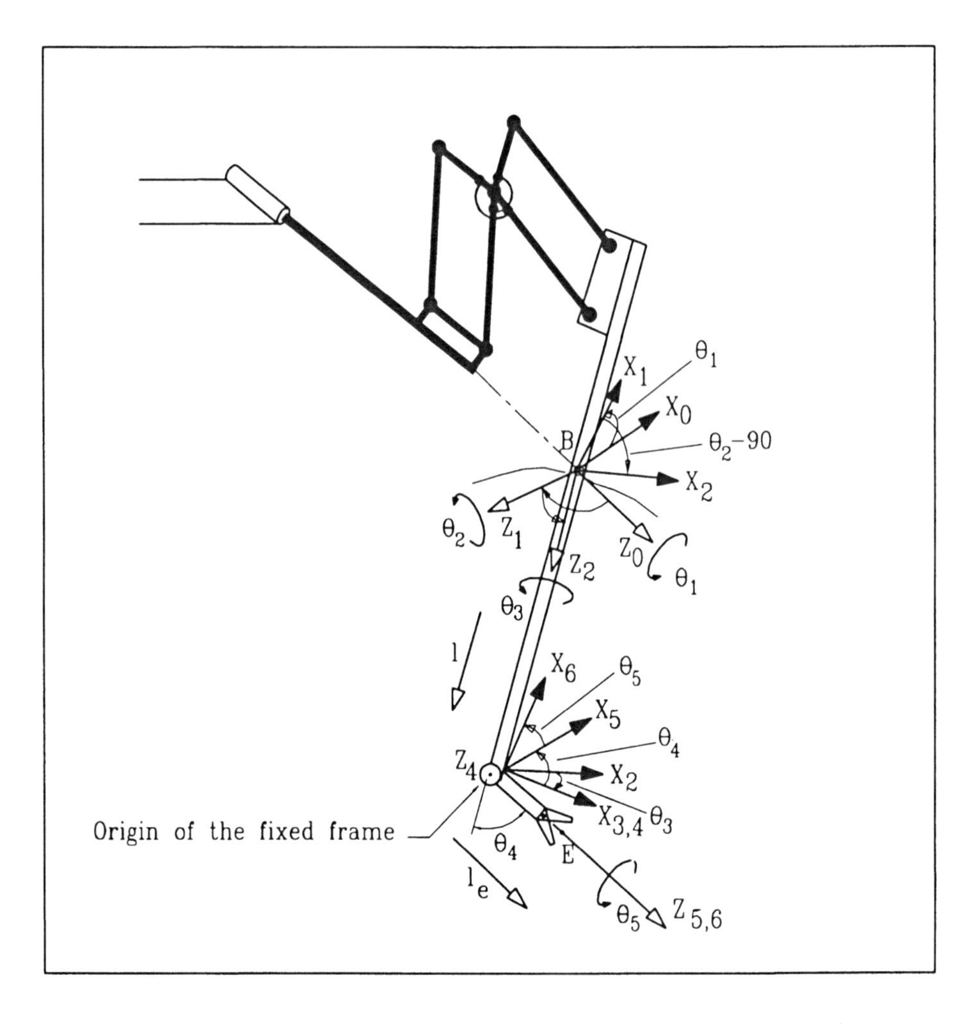

Figure 6.6. Joints coordinate frames of the extender and their transformations.

$$\mathbf{A}_5 = \begin{bmatrix} C_4 & 0 & S_4 & 0 \\ S_4 & 0 & -C_4 & 0 \\ 0 & 1 & 0 & 0 \\ 0 & 0 & 0 & 1 \end{bmatrix} \qquad \mathbf{A}_6 = \begin{bmatrix} C_5 & -S_5 & 0 & 0 \\ S_5 & C_5 & 0 & 0 \\ 0 & 0 & 0 & l_e \\ 0 & 0 & 0 & 1 \end{bmatrix}$$

Therefore, the transformation from the coordinate frame of grasper $\mathbf{X}_6$ to the base frame $\mathbf{X}_0$ at the port of entry (point B, Fig.6.6) would be:

$$\mathbf{X}_0 = \mathbf{A}_1\mathbf{A}_2\mathbf{A}_3\mathbf{A}_4\mathbf{A}_5\mathbf{A}_6\mathbf{X}_6 = \begin{bmatrix} a_{11} & a_{12} & a_{13} & a_{14} \\ a_{21} & a_{22} & a_{23} & a_{24} \\ a_{31} & a_{32} & a_{33} & a_{34} \\ a_{41} & a_{42} & a_{43} & a_{44} \end{bmatrix} \mathbf{X}_6$$

Where,

$$\begin{aligned}
a_{11} &= (C_1S_2C_3 - S_1S_3)C_4C_5 + C_1C_2S_4C_5 - (C_1S_2S_3 + S_1C_3)S_5 \\
a_{21} &= (S_1S_2C_3 + C_1S_3)C_4C_5 + S_1C_2S_4C_5 - (S_1S_2S_3 - C_1C_3)S_5 \\
a_{31} &= C_2C_3C_4C_5 - S_2S_4C_5 - C_2S_3S_5 \\
a_{41} &= 0 \\
a_{12} &= -(C_1S_2C_3 - S_1S_3)C_4S_5 - C_1C_2S_4C_5 - (C_1S_2S_3 + S_1C_3)C_5 \\
a_{22} &= -(S_1S_2C_3 + C_1S_3)C_4S_5 - S_1C_2S_4S_5 - (S_1S_2S_3 - C_1C_3)C_5 \\
a_{32} &= -C_2C_3C_4S_5 + S_2S_4S_5 - C_2S_3C_5 \\
a_{42} &= 0 \\
a_{13} &= (C_1S_2C_3 - S_1S_3)S_4 - C_1C_2C_4 \\
a_{23} &= (S_1S_2C_3 + C_1S_3)S_4 - S_1C_2C_4 \\
a_{33} &= C_2C_3S_4 + S_2C_4 \\
a_{43} &= 0 \\
a_{14} &= (C_1S_2C_3 - S_1S_3)S_4l_e - C_1C_2C_4l_e - C_1C_2l \\
a_{24} &= (S_1S_2C_3 + C_1S_3)S_4l_e - S_1C_2C_4l_e - S_1C_2l \\
a_{34} &= C_2C_3S_4l_e + S_2C_4l_e + S_2l \\
a_{44} &= 1
\end{aligned}$$

And C_i, and S_i are abbreviation of $cos\theta_i$, and $sin\theta_i$ respectively.

The above forward kinematics can be used to obtain the coordinates of the end-point of the laparoscopic extender relative to the base frame $\mathbf{X}_0$ for a known coordinate/configuration of the joints. In addition, the coordinates of other points on any intermediate link/frame (i.e. frames $\mathbf{X}_1$ to $\mathbf{X}_5$) can be obtained relative to the base frame $\mathbf{X}_0$. This can be achieved simply by multiplying the above transformation matrices $A_1A_2....A_n = A$ (where n corresponds to the final intermediate link), which can be used similarly in the forward kinematic equation of $X_0 = AX_n$.

3. JACOBIAN FORMULATION

The kinematics and control related aspects of any robotic manipulator requires the mapping of the velocity between the end-effector (i.e.$[\omega_x, \omega_y, \omega_z, V_x, V_y, V_z]^T$ in the fix base frame $\mathbf{X}_0$) and the velocity of joints ($\dot{\theta}_i$) in the joint coordinate frame, and vice versa. This relationship can be expressed as:

$$\begin{bmatrix} \omega_x \\ \omega_y \\ \omega_z \\ V_x \\ V_y \\ V_z \end{bmatrix} = \mathbf{J} \begin{bmatrix} \dot{\theta_1} \\ \dot{\theta_2} \\ \dot{\theta_3} \\ \dot{l} \\ \dot{\theta_4} \\ \dot{\theta_5} \end{bmatrix} \tag{6.1}$$

where Jacobian **J** is defined as the following matrix:

$$\begin{bmatrix} W_1^x & W_2^x & W_3^x & W_4^x & W_5^x & W_6^x \\ W_1^y & W_2^y & W_3^y & W_4^y & W_5^y & W_6^y \\ W_1^z & W_2^z & W_3^z & W_4^z & W_5^z & W_6^z \\ (W_1 \times r_1)^x & (W_2 \times r_2)^x & (W_3 \times r_3)^x & (W_4 \times r_4)^x & (W_5 \times r_5)^x & (W_6 \times r_6)^x \\ (W_1 \times r_1)^y & (W_2 \times r_2)^y & (W_3 \times r_3)^y & (W_4 \times r_4)^y & (W_5 \times r_5)^y & (W_6 \times r_6)^y \\ (W_1 \times r_1)^z & (W_2 \times r_2)^z & (W_3 \times r_3)^z & (W_4 \times r_4)^z & (W_5 \times r_5)^z & (W_6 \times r_6)^z \end{bmatrix}$$

Where $W_i = [W_i^x, W_i^y, W_i^z]^T$ is a unit vector in the direction of the axis of joint i, and r_i is the vector of the origin of axis i to the reference point of the end-effector[94].

By definition the matrix on the right hand side of Eq.6.1, which acts as a translator between the two velocity states, is called the *Jacobian* of the manipulator[4][78]. In general, determining the Jacobian matrix for a manipulator with high DOF results in two main difficulties as followings:

1. Normally the Jacobian would be a $6 \times N$ matrix (where N is the number of joints or DOF in the manipulator) which creates computational load at each iteration of the incremental movement along the path of trajectory in forward kinematics[2].

2. For inverse kinematics[3], it is even more difficult, since inverting the Jacobian numerically requires intensive computation. This makes real time control of such a manipulator difficult by introducing time delays (due to computational load) or less accurate[4].

Waldron[94] has proposed a novel approach which effectively addresses both of the above difficulties. In summary, the method obtains the Jacobian with simpler terms as elements of the matrix, which can even provide closed-form inverse velocity solution. The two basic key points in this approach are described (by using a simple 3 DOF manipulator

[2]That is finding the velocity state of the end-effector by knowing the velocity state of the joints.

[3]That is finding the velocity state of the joints by knowing the velocity state of the end-effector.

[4]By using point to point approximate routines with less accuracy[78].

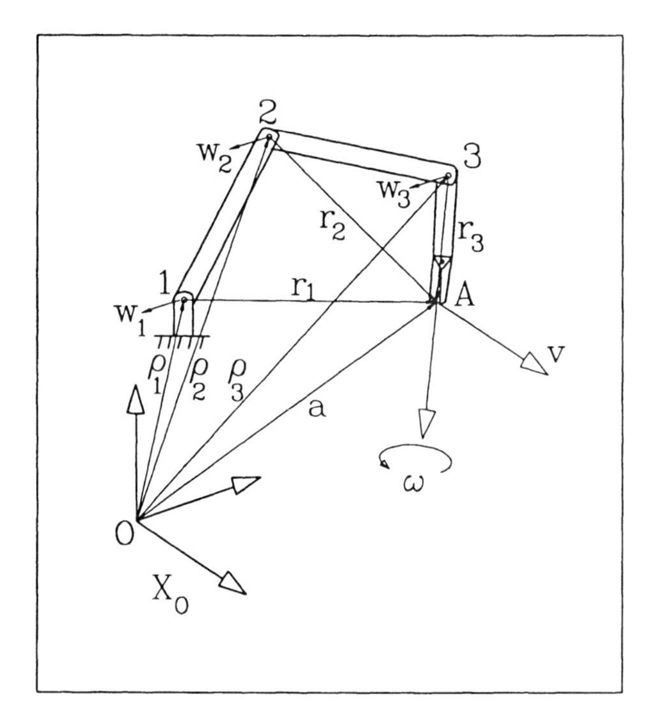

Figure 6.7. Geometric parameters ρ_i and **a** for a 3DOF manipulator.

as an example with a grasper as its end-effector at point A, Fig.6.7) as follows:

- The formulation of Eq. (6.1) is slightly altered, and instead of the velocity $\mathbf{V}$ of the reference point located at the end-effector with respect to the base frame $\mathbf{X}_0$ (Fig.6.7), the velocity μ of a virtual point of the hand instantaneously coincident with the origin (i.e. point O, Fig.6.7) of the fixed frame $\mathbf{X}_0$, is obtained:

$$\mu = \mathbf{V} - \omega \times \mathbf{a} \tag{6.2}$$

  where **a** is the position of the end-effector's reference point (Fig.6.7) relative to the fixed frame $\mathbf{X}_0$, and ω is the angular velocity of the end-effector in that frame.

- To minimize the number of terms in each element of the Jacobian, the fixed frame is transfered to an intermediate link instead of remaining at the base of the manipulator.

In the case of the laparoscopic extender (Fig.6.6), the fixed frame is chosen to be at joint Z_4, and by applying the above formulation[94], the following compact kinematic equation and Jacobian (for detail derivation see App.C) is obtained:

$$\begin{bmatrix} \omega_x \\ \omega_y \\ \omega_z \\ \mu_x \\ \mu_y \\ \mu_z \end{bmatrix} = \begin{bmatrix} C_2C_3 & S_3 & 0 & 0 & 0 & S_4 \\ -S_2 & 0 & -1 & 0 & 0 & -C_4 \\ -C_2S_3 & C_3 & 0 & 0 & 1 & 0 \\ -lC_2S_3 & lC_3 & 0 & 0 & 0 & 0 \\ 0 & 0 & 0 & -1 & 0 & 0 \\ -lC_2C_3 & -lS_3 & 0 & 0 & 0 & 0 \end{bmatrix} \begin{bmatrix} \dot{\theta}_1 \\ \dot{\theta}_2 \\ \dot{\theta}_3 \\ \dot{l} \\ \dot{\theta}_4 \\ \dot{\theta}_5 \end{bmatrix} \tag{6.3}$$

The above equation for forward velocity kinematics is simulated for the full range of motion of all joints (i.e. from coordinates $[-75°, -75°, -180°, 80mm, -120°, -180°]$ to $[75°, 75°, 180°, 280mm, 120°, 180°]$) with constant speed. The constant velocity of each joint is selected so that the full range of travel of the joint would be completed within 10 seconds (Fig. 6.8a to 6.8f, i.e. $\dot{\theta}_1 = \dot{\theta}_2 = 15°/s = 0.262rad/s, \dot{\theta}_3 = \dot{\theta}_5 = 36°/s = 0.628rad/s, \dot{\theta}_4 = 24°/s = 0.419rad/s$, and $\dot{l} = 20mm/s$). The angular velocity of the grasper at the tip of extender (relative to the fix frame $\mathbf{X}_0$, Fig.6.6) is calculated based on Eq.6.3 (Fig.6.8g to i). However, in the case of translational velocity of the grasper (i.e. V_x, V_y, V_z, Fig.6.8j to 6.8L), first the velocity of the virtual point of the grasper at the origin of the base frame (i.e. μ_x, μ_y, μ_z) is calculated by Eq.6.3, then by using Eq.6.2 the velocity of the grasper is calculated as shown in Fig.6.8j to 6.8L.

Having the Jacobian, it is possible to study singularity conditions of the extender. Generally, the manipulator's Jacobian is a function of its configuration, and singularity occurs when the determinant of Jacobian is zero (i.e. $|\mathbf{J}| = 0$), which means the inverse of the Jacobian does not exist at that configuration. Hence at singularity, for bounded velocities of end-effector it requires unbounded joint (s) velocities[4][78], and since this is not possible for any actuator, consequently the manipulator loses at least one of its DOF.

To obtain the determinant, the Jacobian is simplified by its 3rd, 4th, and 5th columns, which yields following further simplifications:

$$|\mathbf{J}| = \begin{vmatrix} C_2C_3 & S_3 & S_4 \\ -lC_2S_3 & lC_3 & 0 \\ -lC_2C_3 & -lS_3 & 0 \end{vmatrix} = l^2C_2S_4 = 0 \tag{6.4}$$

Then singularity occurs when: $l = 0, \theta_2 = \pm 90°, \theta_4 = 0$, and $180°$. However based on the surgical conditions in laparoscopy, the normal range for the parameters[Ch.3] are $l > 80mm$, $-75° < \theta_2 < +75°$, and

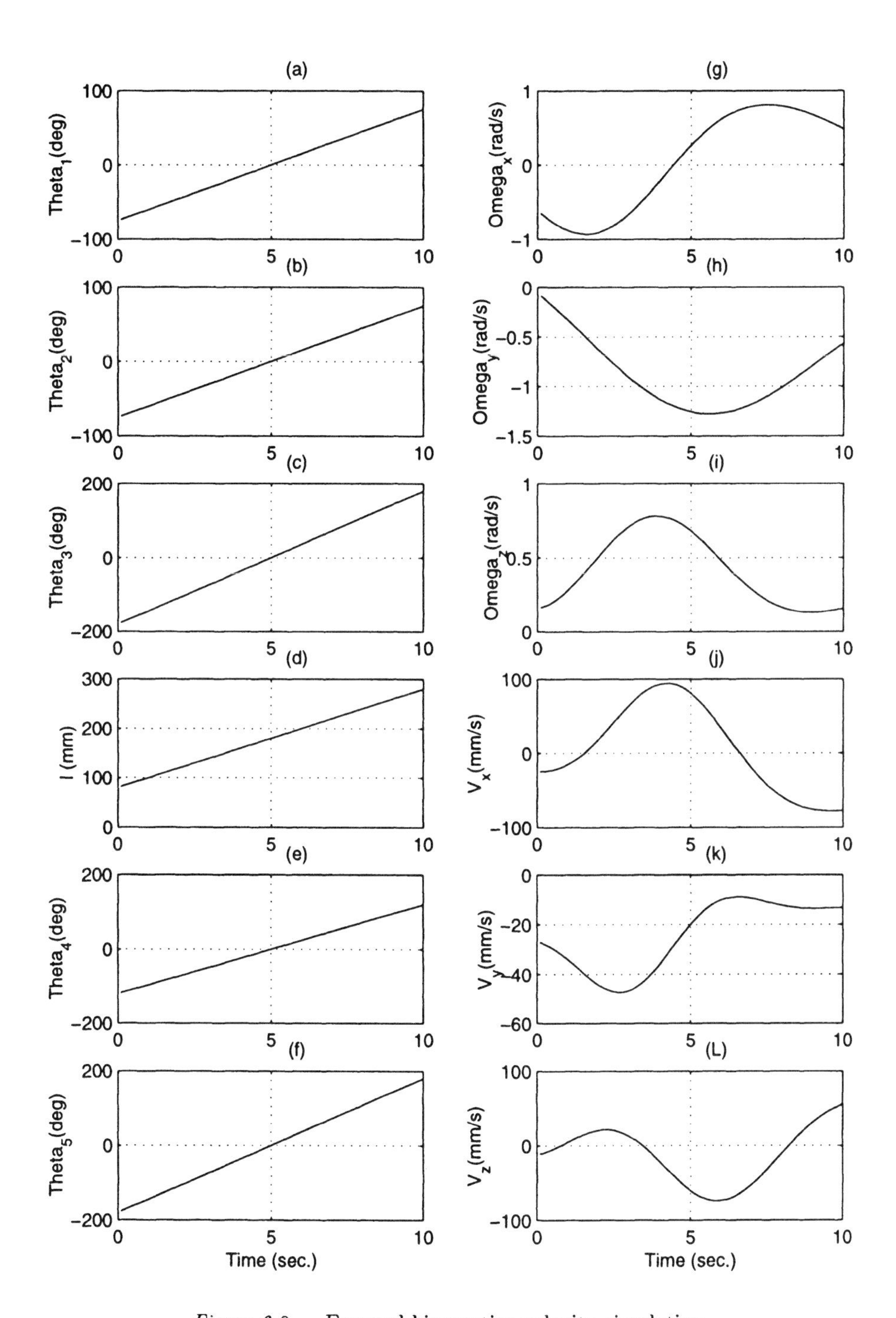

Figure 6.8. Forward kinematics velocity simulation.

$-120° \leq \theta_4 \leq 120°$. Therefore, the only possibility for the occurrence of singularity is when $\theta_4 = 0$. This is the case when the shank of the flexible stem is fully straight without any bend, and the axes Z_3, and Z_5 are collinear (Fig. 6.6). This means, at the singularity, the manipulator loses 1 DOF in dexterity (of orienting the grasper toward the surgical site). To avoid the singularity, then $\theta_4 \neq 0$ must be satisfied, and for dexterous operation of the extender θ_4 should not approach the zero value but remain in a higher range (e.g. $\theta_4 > 30°$).

4. INVERSE VELOCITY KINEMATICS

The compact formulation of velocity relationship (Eq.6.3) makes it possible to solve analytically for the joints' velocity in terms of the defined end-point velocity. Re-arranging equations we have:

$$\begin{cases} C_2C_3\dot{\theta}_1 + S_3\dot{\theta}_2 + S_4\dot{\theta}_5 &= \omega_x \\ -S_2\dot{\theta}_1 - \dot{\theta}_3 - C_4\dot{\theta}_5 &= \omega_y \\ -C_2S_3\dot{\theta}_1 + C_3\dot{\theta}_2 + \dot{\theta}_4 &= \omega_z \\ -lC_2S_3\dot{\theta}_1 + lC_3\dot{\theta}_2 &= \mu_x \\ -\dot{l} &= \mu_y \\ -lC_2C_3\dot{\theta}_1 - lS_3\dot{\theta}_2 &= \mu_z \end{cases}$$

Or solving for the joint velocities:

$$\begin{cases} \dot{\theta}_1 &= -(S_3\mu_x + C_3\mu_z)/lC_2 \\ \dot{\theta}_2 &= (C_3\mu_x - S_3\mu_z)/l \\ \dot{\theta}_3 &= -(C_4/S_4)\omega_x - \omega_y + (S_2S_3/lC_2)\mu_x - (C_4/lS_4 - C_3S_2/lC_2)\mu_z \\ \dot{l} &= -\mu_y \\ \dot{\theta}_4 &= \omega_z - \mu_x/l \\ \dot{\theta}_5 &= (\omega_x + \mu_z/l)/S_4 \end{cases}$$

Which can be written in the inverse formulation $\dot{\theta} = \mathbf{J}^{-1}\dot{X}$ as:

$$\begin{bmatrix} \dot{\theta}_1 \\ \dot{\theta}_2 \\ \dot{\theta}_3 \\ \dot{l} \\ \dot{\theta}_4 \\ \dot{\theta}_5 \end{bmatrix} = \begin{bmatrix} 0 & 0 & 0 & -\frac{S_3}{lC_2} & 0 & -\frac{C_3}{lC_2} \\ 0 & 0 & 0 & \frac{C_3}{l} & 0 & -\frac{S_3}{l} \\ \frac{-C_4}{S_4} & -1 & 0 & \frac{S_2S_3}{lC_2} & 0 & -(\frac{C_4}{lS_4} - \frac{S_2C_3}{lC_2}) \\ 0 & 0 & 0 & 0 & -1 & 0 \\ 0 & 0 & 1 & -\frac{1}{l} & 0 & 0 \\ \frac{1}{S_4} & 0 & 0 & 0 & 0 & \frac{1}{lS_4} \end{bmatrix} \begin{bmatrix} \omega_x \\ \omega_y \\ \omega_z \\ \mu_x \\ \mu_y \\ \mu_z \end{bmatrix} \quad (6.5)$$

The above equation is simulated by using the motion of endpoint (i.e.$[\omega, \mu]$)from the previous simulation (i.e. Eq.6.3), as the input for

Eq.6.5. The virtue of doing so is to verify if the inverse velocity kinematics can indeed reproduce the initial constant speeds used as input to the forward kinematics (i.e. Eq.6.3, Fig.6.8a to 6.8f). As shown in Fig.6.9g to 6.9L, the output of inverse kinematic velocity (Eq.6.5) is identical to the input of forward kinematic velocity (Fig.6.8a to 6.8f), with the only difference that, at $t = 5sec.$, where $\theta_4 = 0$, for bounded input, the output values of $\dot{\theta}_3$, and $\dot{\theta}_5$ are unbounded (Fig.6.9i and 6.9L at t=5sec.). This is caused by the singularity at $\theta_4 = 0$, when the two axes θ_3, and θ_5 are collinear, and the extender loses 1 DOF in angular motion at the end-point.

The above inverse kinematic equation can be used for *resolved motion rate control* [4][96], or calculating instantaneous incremental movements of the grasper in real time for point to point trajectory path control.

5. CONSTRAINED MOTION

Robotic manipulators usually have to work with specific motion constraints which reduce their total number of DOF[78]. For example, to perform the task of painting on a flat surface, the end-effector has to move in an equidistant plane parallel to the painting surface and have a normal orientation toward the plane, and in welding not only has the end-effector to follow the exact path of the seam, it also has to remain at a specific orientation with respect to the seam.

In laparoscopy, there are constrained motions such as manipulation of tissue at the surgical site. In this case, basically the surgeon grasps the tissue with the extender, then changes its orientation while the position of the grasping point should remain the same in order to prevent any undesired pull or tear of the tissue (Fig.6.10). This constrained motion requires freedom of movement in orienting the extender, while its tip has a *fixed position* in the work space (Fig.6.10).

On the other hand, there is another type of constrained motion in laparoscopy related to tasks that require *fixed orientation*, such as suturing. In this task, the needle should penetrate the tissue while its orientation should remain the same (with respect to the fixed work space coordinate frame XYZ, Fig.6.11).

In the following sections, the kinematics of extender and the mapping of its joints movements based on the two types of constrained motions described above (i.e. fixed position, and fixed orientation) are analyzed and discussed.

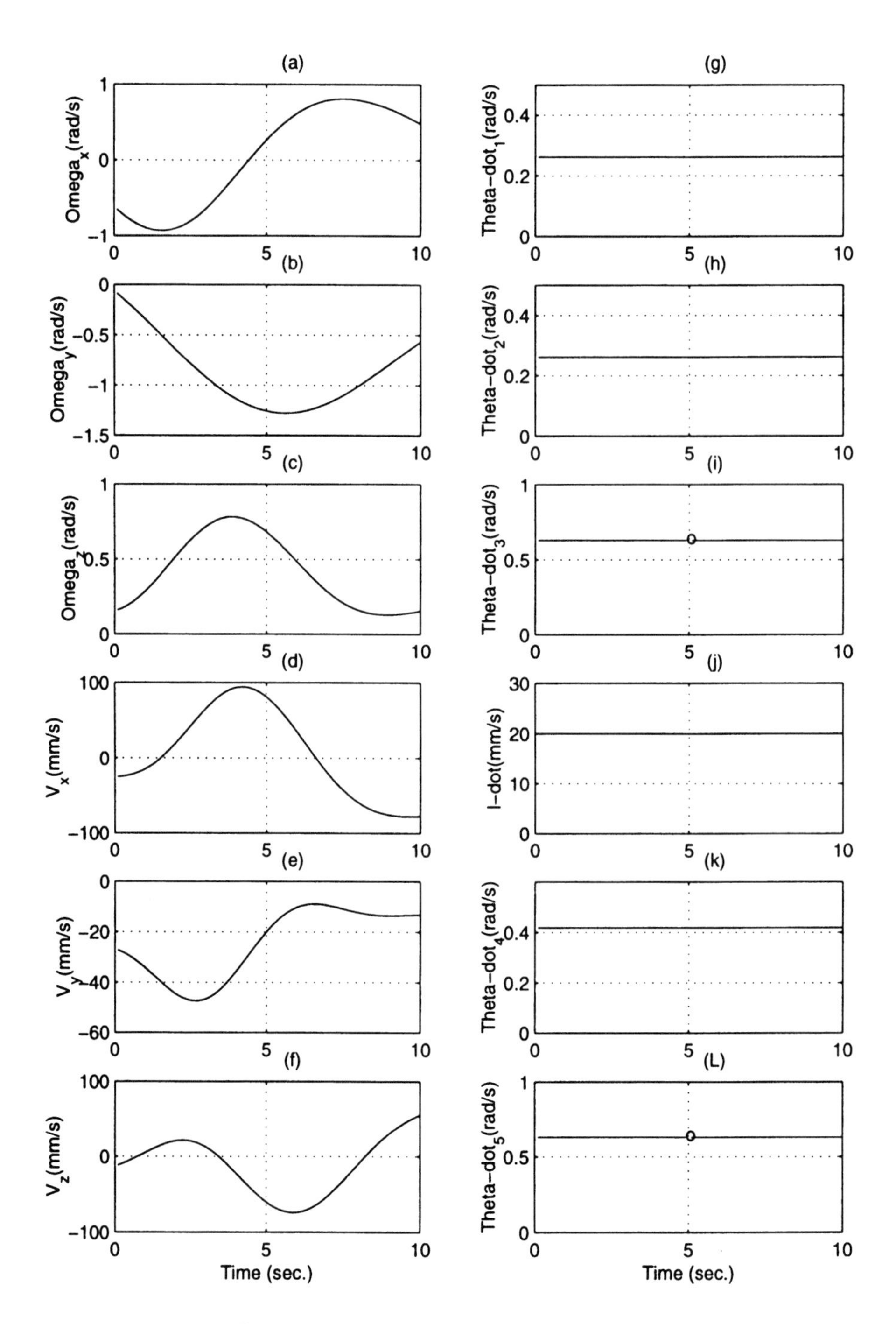

Figure 6.9. Inverse kinematics simulation.

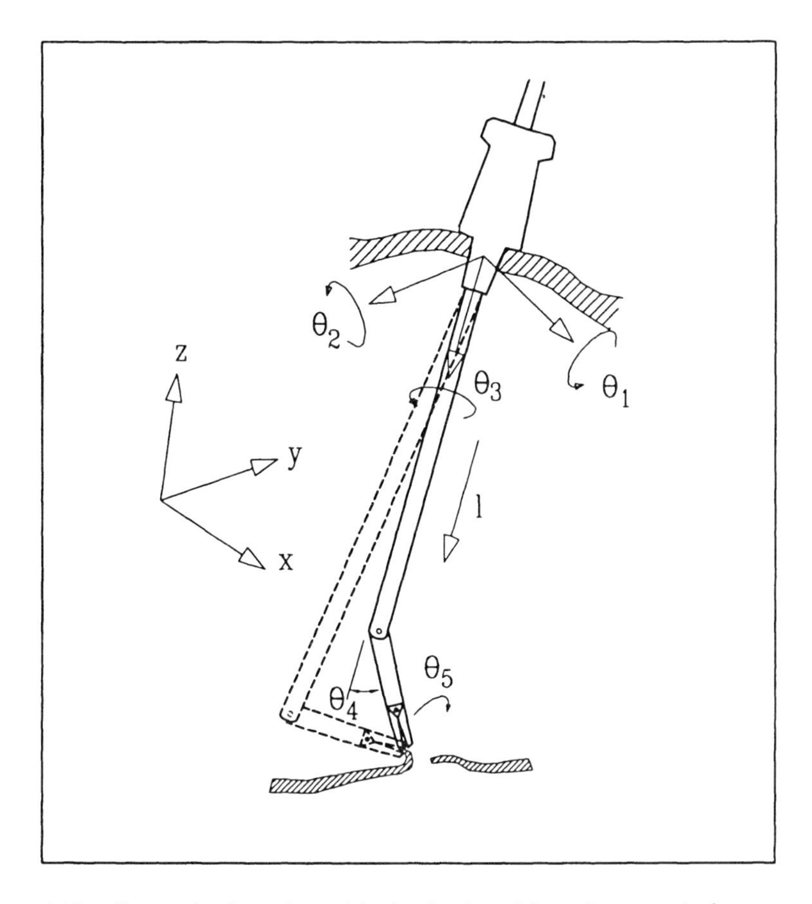

Figure 6.10. Constrained motion with the fixed position of grasper in laparoscopy.

5.1 FIXED POSITION CONSTRAINT

This constraint requires the angular velocity vector of grasper ω to vary, while its velocity vector $\mathbf{V}$ remains zero. Hence, by using Eq.6.2, $\mathbf{V} = \mu + \omega \times \mathbf{a}$, and substituting $\mathbf{a} = [l_e S_4, -l_e C_4, 0]^T$ (i.e. the position vector of the grasper with respect to the fixed coordinate frame $\mathbf{X}_0$), as well as μ and ω obtained from Eq.6.3, we would have:

$$\mathbf{V} = \begin{bmatrix} -lC_2S_3\dot{\theta}_1 + lC_3\dot{\theta}_2 \\ -\dot{l} \\ -lC_2C_3\dot{\theta}_1 - lS_3\dot{\theta}_2 \end{bmatrix} + \begin{bmatrix} C_2C_3\dot{\theta}_1 + S_3\dot{\theta}_2 + S_4\dot{\theta}_5 \\ -S_2\dot{\theta}_1 - \dot{\theta}_3 - C_4\dot{\theta}_5 \\ -C_2S_3\dot{\theta}_1 + C_3\dot{\theta}_2 + \dot{\theta}_4 \end{bmatrix} \times \begin{bmatrix} l_eS_4 \\ -l_eC_4 \\ 0 \end{bmatrix} = \begin{bmatrix} 0 \\ 0 \\ 0 \end{bmatrix}$$

This leads us to the following constraint equations:

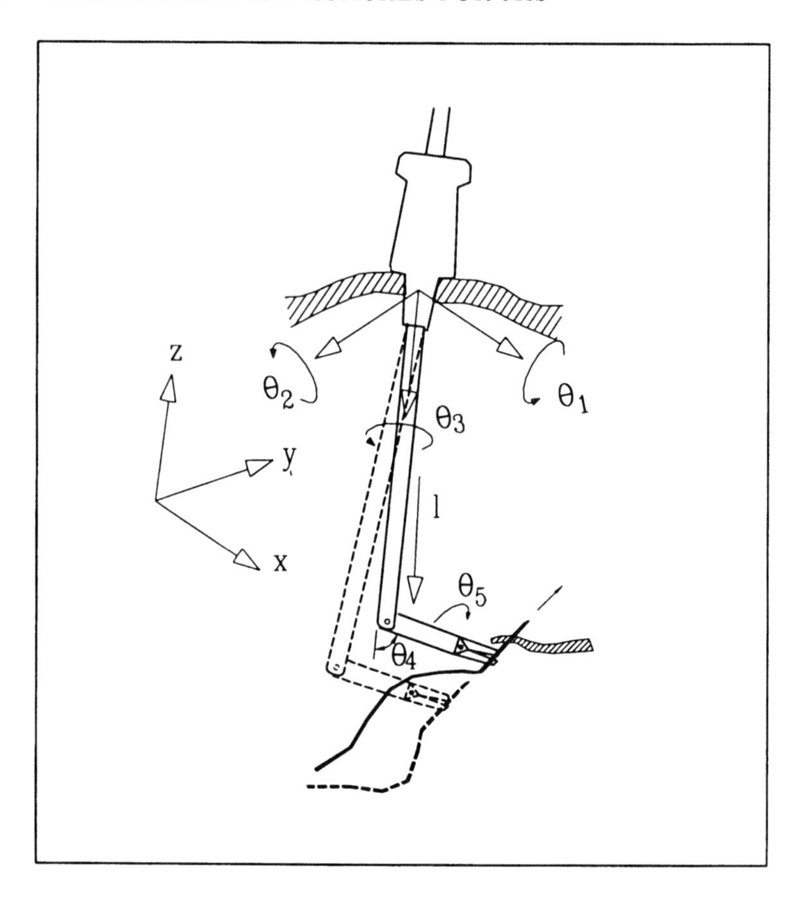

Figure 6.11. Constrained motion with the fixed orientation of grasper in laparoscopy.

$$\begin{cases} (l + l_e C_4)(-C_2 S_3 \dot{\theta}_1 + C_3 \dot{\theta}_2) + l_e C_4 \dot{\theta}_4 = 0 \\ -\dot{l} + l_e S_4(-C_2 S_3 \dot{\theta}_1 + C_3 \dot{\theta}_2 + \dot{\theta}_4) = 0 \\ (l C_2 C_3 + l_e C_2 C_3 C_4 - l_e S_2 S_4)\dot{\theta}_1 + S_3(l + l_e C_4)\dot{\theta}_2 - (l_e S_4)\theta_3 = 0 \end{cases}$$

The above equations can be solved for any set of three variables from the 5 joints variables (i.e. $\dot{\theta}_1, \dot{\theta}_2, \dot{\theta}_3, \dot{\theta}_4$, and $\dot{l}$) as a function of other remaining 2 variables. However, since the constraints here are related to the fixed position of grasper, we select the positioning axes (i.e. θ_1, θ_2, and l, that carry out the positioning of the laparoscopic grasper at the surgical site) of the extender to be function (or slave) of the orienting axes (i.e. θ_3, and θ_4, that orient the tip of the grasper at the surgical site) as follows:

$$\dot{\theta}_1 = \frac{l_e(S_4 C_3 \dot{\theta}_3 + S_3 C_4 \dot{\theta}_4)}{C_2(l + l_e C_4) - l_e S_2 C_3 S_4} \tag{6.6}$$

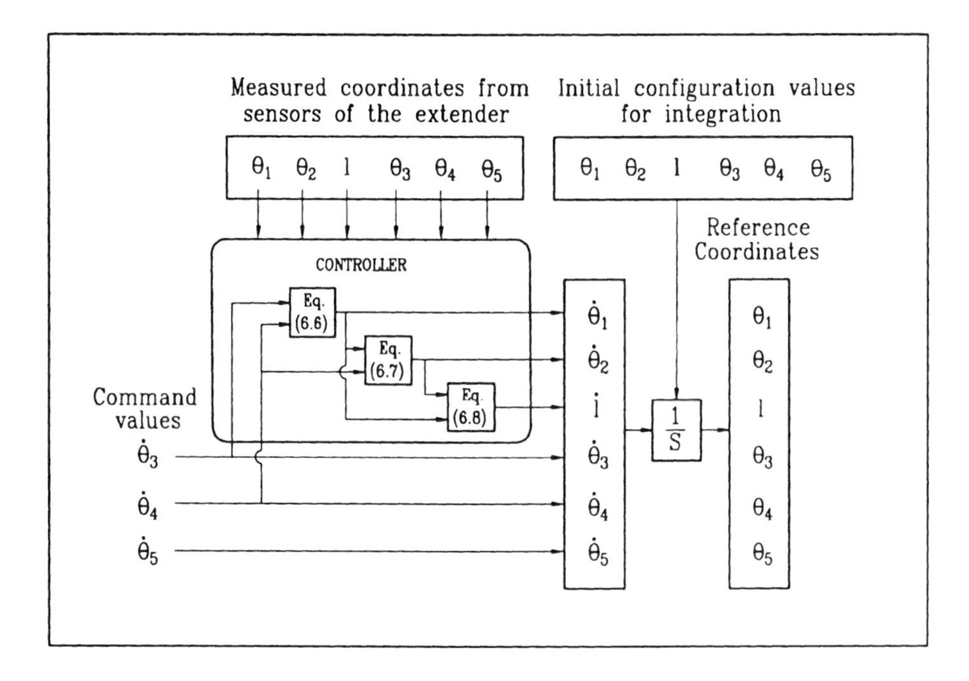

Figure 6.12. Block diagram of fixed position controller.

$$\dot{\theta}_2 = \frac{-l_e C_4}{C_3(l + l_e C_4)}\dot{\theta}_4 + \frac{C_2 S_3}{C_3}\dot{\theta}_1 \tag{6.7}$$

$$\dot{l} = \frac{l.l_e S_4}{l + l_e C_4}\dot{\theta}_4 \tag{6.8}$$

For control purposes of the laparoscopic extender, it is possible to use the above equations when the *fixed position* constraint is desirable for manipulation of tissues (Fig.6.12). In this case the surgeon can switch the controller to the mode shown by the block diagram Fig.6.12, so that the positioning axes (i.e. θ_1, θ_2, and l) are controlled by orienting axes (i.e. θ_3, and θ_4) as slave axes automatically. Hence, the surgeon can control only the desired axes which in this case are orienting axes (i.e. θ_3, and θ_4), while the fixed position of the tip of the extender is assured by the controller (Fig.6.12).

The *fixed position* constraint is simulated while joints θ_3, and θ_4 are moving as the orienting axes, with constant angular velocities of $\dot{\theta}_3 = \dot{\theta}_5 = 9°/s = 0.157 rad/s, \dot{\theta}_4 = 5°/s = 0.0873 rad/s$, from initial coordinate of $[-75°, -75°, -180°, 80mm, -120°, -180°]$ to $[0°, 0°, 0°, 200mm, 20°, 0°]$. By using Eq.6.6, 6.7, and 6.8, the velocities of other three slave positioning axes (i.e. $\dot{\theta}_1, \dot{\theta}_2$, and $\dot{l}$) have been calculated for every time increment of 0.01 second. However, it must be pointed out that at each new time increment, the coordinate θ_2 is initially unknown in equations 6.6, and 6.7. Therefore, in the first iteration, the coordinate θ_2 of previous time increment is used as a first approximation, in order to calculate $\dot{\theta}_2$. Then, in the second iteration, θ_2 is calculated by integration of the obtained $\dot{\theta}_2$ (from the previous iteration) over the time increment of 0.01sec. After only two iterations, the calculated joint slave velocities $[\dot{\theta}_1, \dot{\theta}_2, \dot{l}]$ converge to such a tolerance that the obtained fix position constraint of the end point is satisfied to the level that its movement in any direction is less than 1.3 micrometer (the maximum error by moving in different directions are $\Delta x = -0.43$, $\Delta y = -0.12$, and $\Delta z = -1.2$ micrometer) for the full range of the above simulated motion. The result of holding the tool tip stationary by the controller while its orientation is continuously changed is quite satisfactory by this method, and shows the equations 6.6 to 6.8 can provide the desired fixed position constraint by simple iterative algorithms (such as the above routine).

5.2 FIXED ORIENTATION CONSTRAINT

In this case, the angular velocity vector of extender ω should remain zero, while the grasper is moving in the work space. Hence, by using ω from Eq.6.3 and equating it to zero, we obtain:

$$\begin{cases} \omega_x = 0 = C_2C_3\dot{\theta}_1 + S_3\dot{\theta}_2 + S_4\dot{\theta}_5 \\ \omega_y = 0 = -S_2\dot{\theta}_1 - \dot{\theta}_3 - C_4\dot{\theta}_5 \\ \omega_z = 0 = -C_2S_3\dot{\theta}_1 + C_3\dot{\theta}_2 + \dot{\theta}_4 \end{cases}$$

The orientation of the tip of the grasper is controlled by joints θ_3, θ_4, and θ_5 near the surgical site. Hence, the above constraint equations are solved for the orienting axes θ_3, θ_4, and θ_5 as a function of positioning axes θ_1, and θ_2 of the extender as follows:

$$\dot{\theta}_3 = -C_4\dot{\theta}_5 - S_2\dot{\theta}_1 = (S_3\dot{\theta}_2 + C_2C_3\dot{\theta}_1)C_4/S_4 - S_2\dot{\theta}_1 \tag{6.9}$$

$$\dot{\theta}_4 = -C_3\dot{\theta}_2 + C_2S_3\dot{\theta}_1 \tag{6.10}$$

$$\dot{\theta}_5 = -(S_3\dot{\theta}_2 + C_2C_3\dot{\theta}_1)/S_4 \tag{6.11}$$

The above equations can be used to implement the *fixed orientation* constraint by using the control mode shown in the block diagram (Fig.6.14), so that the orienting axes (i.e. θ_3, and θ_4) are controlled by positioning axes (i.e.θ_1, and θ_2) as slave axes automatically. Hence, the surgeon can control only the desired axes which in this case are positioning axes (i.e. θ_3, and θ_4) to move the tip of the extender to any desired coordinate near the surgical site, while the fixed orientation of the grasper is assured by the controller (Fig.6.14).

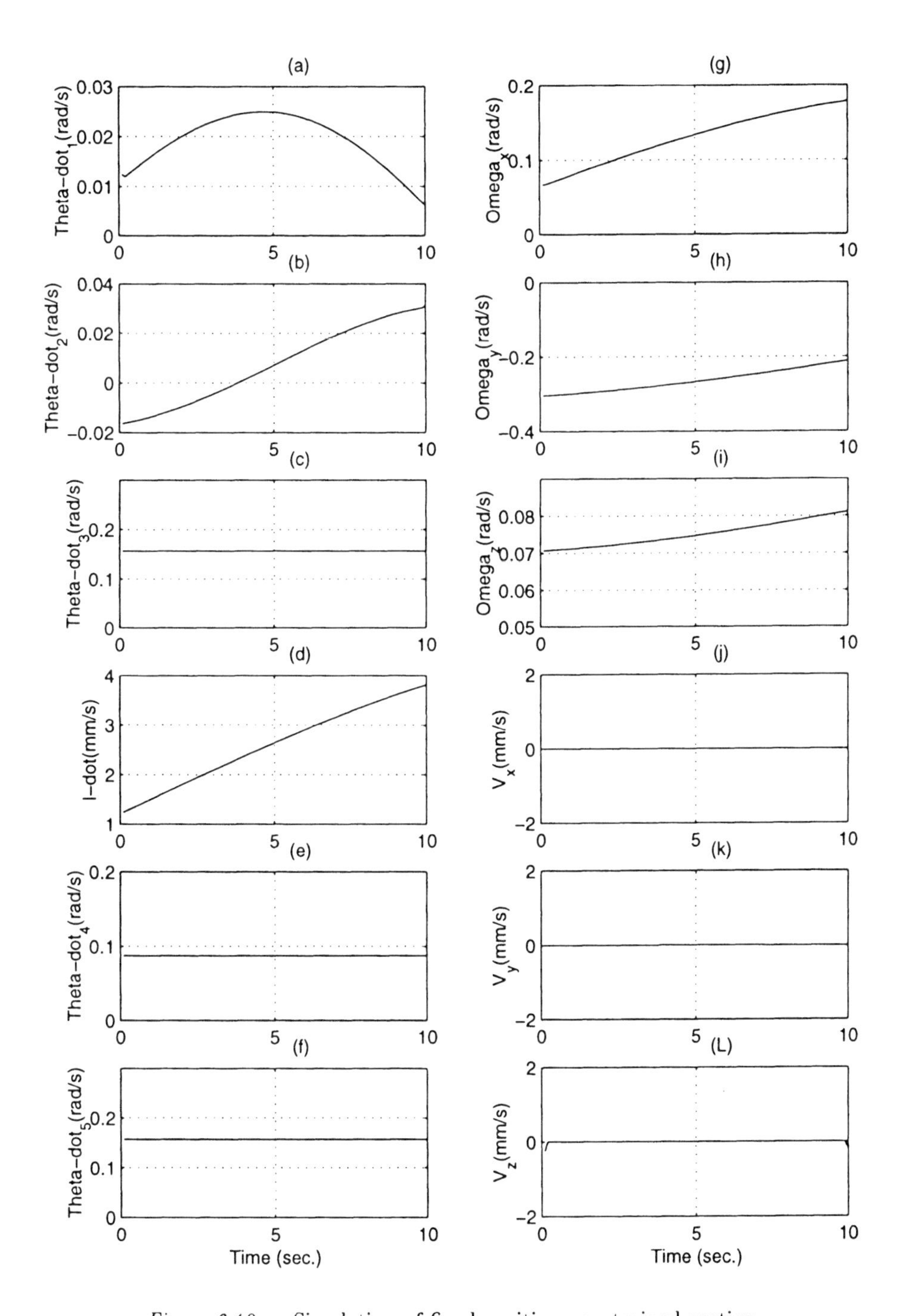

Figure 6.13. Simulation of fixed position constrained motion.

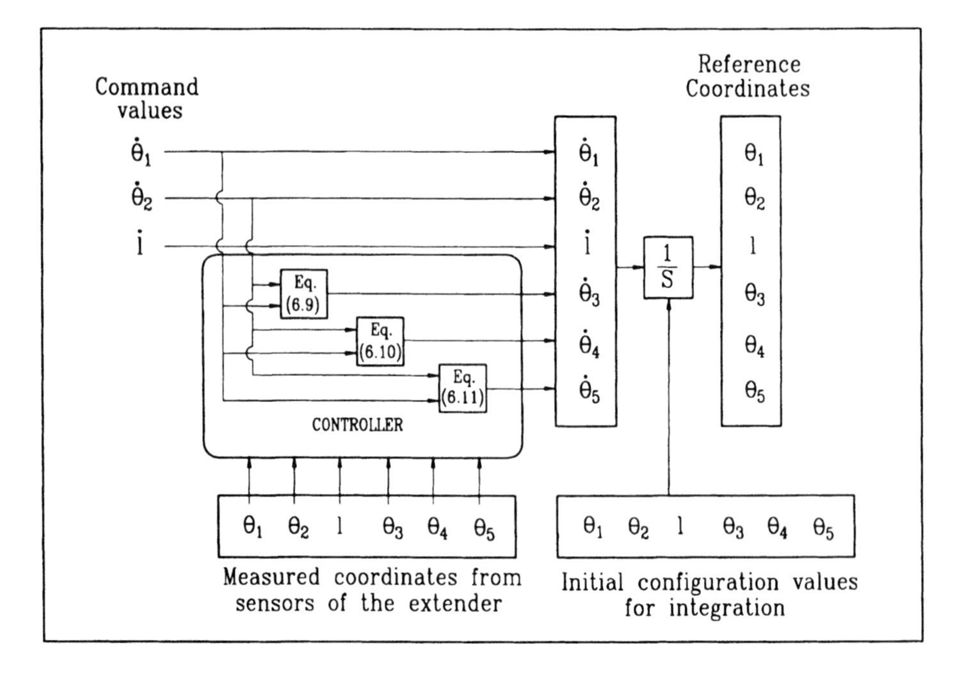

Figure 6.14. Block diagram of fixed orientation controller.

This is simulated similarly by generating constant joint velocities for positioning axes (i.e. $\dot{\theta}_1 = \dot{\theta}_2 = 9°/s = 0.157 rad/s$, Fig.6.15). The initial value of θ_4 for Eq.6.9 is obtained from the previous time increment, then after obtaining $\dot{\theta}_4$, it is integrated over time increment of 0.01 sec. to obtain θ_4 for the second iteration. After 4 iterations of $\dot{\theta}_3, \dot{\theta}_4$, and $\dot{\theta}_5$, the joints coordinates converge to such a tolerance that the fixed orientation constraint is satisfied to less than a tenth of degree for the full range of movement, Fig.6.15 (the maximum angular movements around different axes are $\Delta\theta_x = 0.071°, \Delta\theta_y = 0.001°$, and $\Delta\theta_z = 0.074°$).

6. TOWARD LAPAROSCOPIC TELE-SURGERY

The main difficulty in laparoscopy is the usage of very long tools through fixed small incision points. No matter how much the design of tool (both in terms of degrees of freedom and optimum interface with the surgeon's hand) is improved, still direct physical hand control of the tool is unnatural, remote, and physically demanding. Only with training and practice, it is possible for the surgeon to obtain a fraction of the skill level of open surgery. To improve dexterity to the level comparable to open surgery, direct hand control of laparoscopic tools can not be the solution. As a result, further improvement lies in the development of

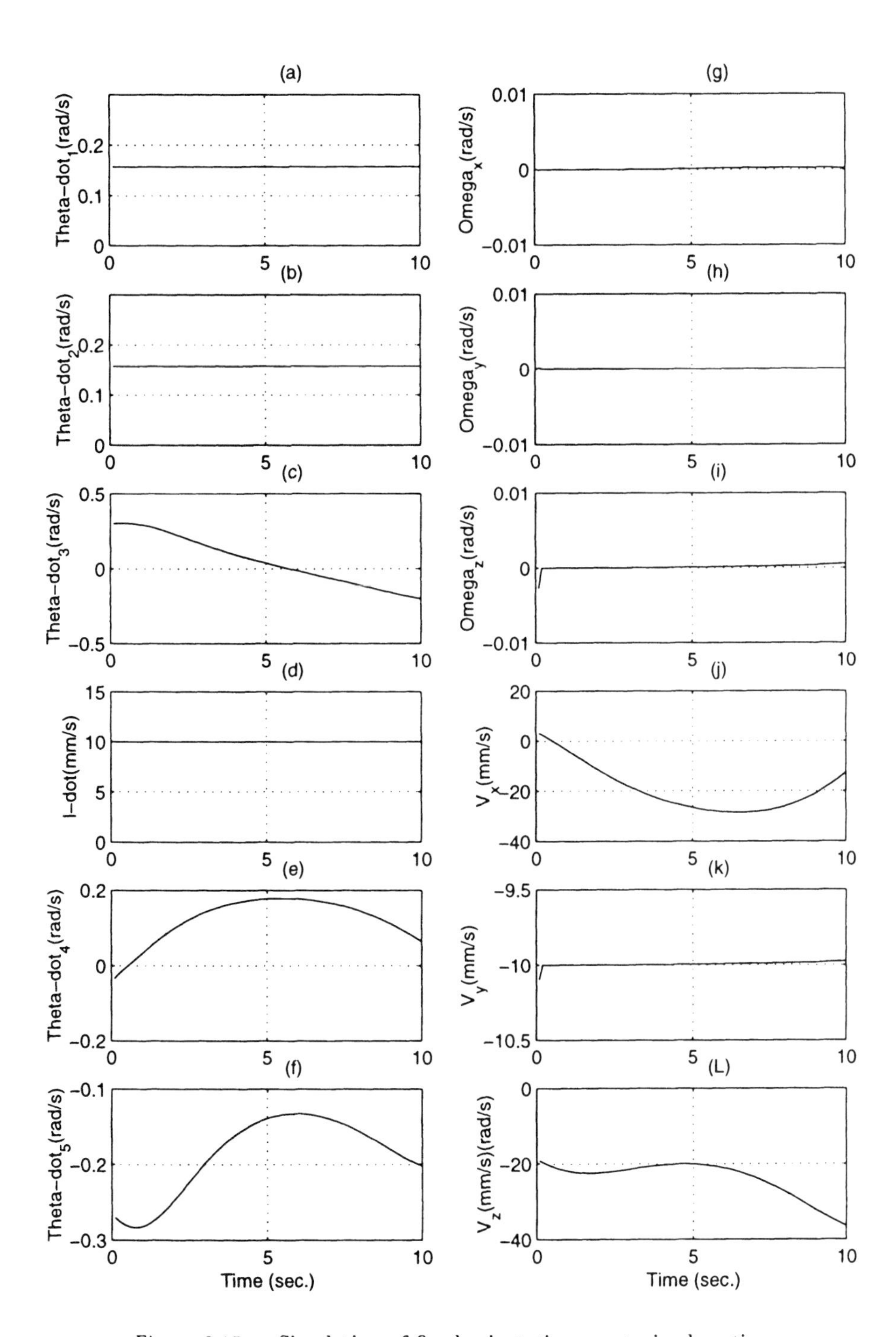

Figure 6.15. Simulation of fixed orientation constrained motion.

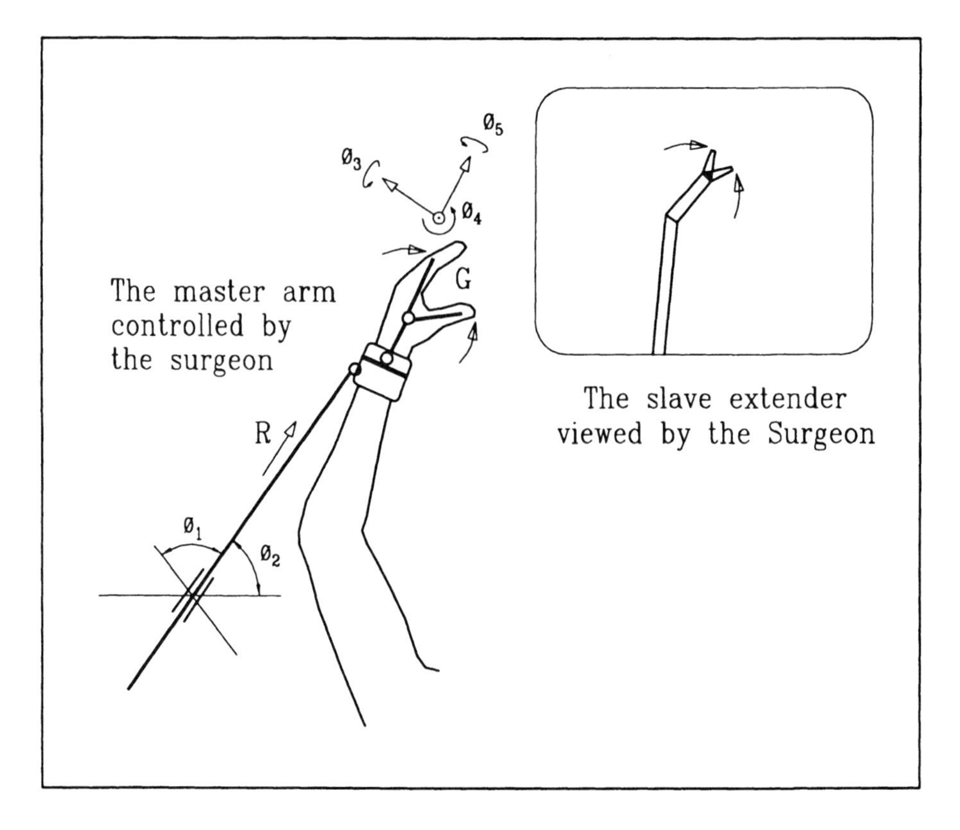

Figure 6.16. Schematics of the master arm.

robotic extenders (e.g. Fig.6.4) which can be indirectly controlled by the surgeon through a master arm (Fig.6.16). This master-slave robotic system controls the movements of the robotic extender inside the abdominal cavity, which is controlled indirectly by hand movements of the surgeon on a tele-surgical workstation[32].

The success of such a system not only depends on the general control characteristics of the master-slave system (such as accuracy, fast response, and force reflection [8] [76]), but also its ease of usage by the surgeon. For example to control the extender by means of a "joystick" type of design is not a natural interface for the surgeon, since all the end-effectors movements would have to be translated to movements of the joystick by logical step by step reasoning, instead of subconscious natural control.

Based on the kinematic study of robotic extenders for laparoscopy, and the above motivation for tele-operation, the following is a proposed master/slave configuration subject of future detail design and development.

The Slave : The slave extenders (Fig.6.4) with 6 DOF can be mounted on the arms of a positioning stand similar to the one synthesized in Ch. 2 . The positioning stand in this case is a passive mechanism that holds the extenders in the proper position and orientation with respect to the incision points.

The Master : In order to achieve an easy to control master-slave system, which does not require substantial training, it is essential for the slave to mimic hand movements. This means the mechanical movements of the extender should be mapped and controlled by natural movements of human hand. There could be various alternative configurations for the master arm. The key point in the design configuration of the master arm are:

1. The angular orientation of the hand based on the 3 DOF of the wrist to be measured as coordinates ϕ_3, ϕ_4, and ϕ_5 by the master (Fig.6.16), which are mapped to coordinates θ_3, θ_4, and θ_5 of the slave extender (Fig.6.4) respectively.
2. The positioning coordinate of the hand to be measured (i.e. ϕ_1, ϕ_2, and R), and then mapped to the positioning coordinates of the extender (i.e. θ_1, θ_2, and l).
3. The grasping action of extender to be sensed directly by the angular motion of the thumb G, with respect to other fingers and being reflected directly to the grasper (Fig.6.16).

Force reflection is an important sensing and safety issue that could be incorporated into the master-slave system. This could be achieved by using bilateral tele-operation schemes (e.g. bilateral position control proposed by Becquet[8]), which requires future developments for the laparoscopic applications. Though bandwidth and accuracy of reflection are pending matters for further research along the previous works[45] [72][97] in bilateral tele-operation systems.

Chapter 7

CONCLUSIONS

1. CONTRIBUTIONS OF THE BOOK

This study has led us into diverse fields of research, which is a natural part of robotics research. Though it was not possible to pursue all of them, the ones studied provided us with a number of contributions which are categorized based on each type of development as follows:

I - Positioning Stand : The positioning stand is a new approach [23] [29] [32] in providing external support for the surgeon by using a passive mechanism in order to improve her/his dexterity, performance, and reducing the physical stress compared to the current passive arms [2] used only for locking tools. The positioning stand as a patented mechanism[26] has the following main contributing features:

1. **New wrist mechanism:**

   This mechanism simulates exactly the movements of a spherical joint located at the port of entry. This is the first application of such a concentric multi-link spherical joint[23][26][28] for laparoscopic systems, although it had been proposed for other applications such as space-frames[43]. Other parallelogram mechanisms proposed by other research groups [49][86] , are actually a special case of the concentric multi-link spherical joint[23][28]. The general aspect of this design provides more design variables(i.e. ϕ, and l_3, Chapter 2), which allows to be optimized and miniaturized into more compact wrist mechanism with less space requirement, which is crucial for laparoscopy.

2. **New modular arm design:**

   This comprises of a multi-arm system, mounted on a column structure, to provide support for each of the wrist mechanisms. This is a flexible modular system that allows the number of arms, their location, and configuration to be varied/adjusted, as well as being able to lock them pneumatically based on the surgical requirements of the specific procedure[23][26][28].

<u>**II - Dexterous Extenders :**</u> This study has led us to three designs of flexible stems[32][25]. After comparative analysis and development(Ch.3), the following contributions can be concluded:

3. **Single joint flexible stem with 4 bar-linkage actuation:**

   This is a robust and dexterous design with the total joint rotation up to 120° which is implemented as laparoscopic graspers for the first time[25]. This design provides ample flexibility of the stem, while providing access to the end of the extender for actuation/sensing of the grasper. The design provides up to 2 additional DOF inside the abdomen to rotate the tool's tip, and can readily be implemented on manual hand-held tools, as well as on actuated robotic extenders(Ch.6).

4. **Multi-Spherical joints flexible stem with tendons actuation:**

   It has been analyzed[30] and experimentally prototyped to demonstrate its potential of providing up to 3 DOF to rotate the tool's tip inside the body. Analysis has shown this type of flexible joint has the highest range of dexterity[25], however the actuation of joints by tendons is relatively more complicated to implement and control.

5. **New measure of dexterity for laparoscopy:**

   The newly defined global dexterity measure is an effective way to compare dexterous workspaces of different laparoscopic extenders with flexible stems within their reachable workspace[25]. The measure of dexterity(Eq.3.1) can also be used generally for manipulators or robots in a planar formulation to access their dexterity.

6. **New mathematical model for joints friction:**

   Mathematical models for the frictional moment at spherical/revolute joints [30](App.A) have been developed analytically for the purpose of actuation/locking of joints, as well as motion control of both revolute or spherical joints. This is a general mathematical analysis with the realistic assumption of non-rigidity of the joint material, which yields a more accurate model than the simple assumption of the absolute rigidity of the joints. The models are in simple closed forms which could have numerous applications in the design of mechanisms, the control aspects of multi-body systems, and robotics.

III - Automated Devices: In the field of automated suturing and knotting, there has been contributions both in a new developmental design which led to a patent[24], as well as miniaturization aspects:

7. **New class of suturing device:**

   This new class of suturing device[32] is based on circular motion of needle that could be used in laparoscopy as well as open surgery[24] to perform the suturing task.

8. **Knotting by the suturing device:**

   The knotting task was not considered in the scope of the suturing device at the design stage, however, by using the technique proposed in Chapter 4, without needing a separate knotting device, it is possible to perform the knotting task semi-automatically in much shorter time with relative ease compared to the manual knotting.

IV - Force Reflection : For haptic interface and force reflection to the hand of surgeon from laparoscopic graspers[32], the following contributions have been made:

9. **Force Reflecting Grasper:**

   The design and experimental implementation of a force-reflecting grasper for laparoscopy[1][22][33] by using the tunable spring as a passive variable stiffness, is a new approach to reflect/regulate haptic forces[27].

10. **Controller for Spring Actuation:**

    The design of appropriate control laws which regulate the tunable spring by controlling both the transmission ratio from handle to grasper and the maximum level of grasping force [1][22] [33].

11. **General Applications in Haptic Interfacing:**

    The above approach of tunable spring and its controller can have further contributions beyond the specific domain of laparoscopy[27].

The contributions can be in any linkage mechanism where decoupling of *kinematics* (motion transmission) and *kinetics* (force transmission) is a design goal, or a functional requirement for controlled transmission of forces.

V - Robotics : In the field of robotic applications for Minimally Invasive Surgery (e.g. laparoscopy[32]), there are contributions in the design configuration of robotic extenders, as well as kinematic analysis of such robotic extenders as follows:

12. **Configuration of Robotic Extenders for Laparoscopy:**

    The design configuration of laparoscopic robotic extenders with 4 DOF for automated positioning applications, as well as extenders with up to 6 DOF for dexterous extenders in tele-operated applications have been studied.

13. **Kinematics of the Robotic Extenders:**

    The kinematic and singularity study of the robotic extenders, as well as the constrained motion analysis, has provided us with constrained equations of motion of joints. These equations can be used for the automatic controlled motion of joints to obtain the desired constrained motion.

2. SUGGESTIONS FOR FUTURE WORK

There are many open avenues in each of the previously mentioned fields, so research about laparoscopic tools and systems can be continued, resulting in numerous types of different developments. However, based on the outcome of this research, there are some suggestions which are either the next logical step of previously mentioned developments, or have potentials for new developmental works, as follows:

I - Single Modular Positioning Arms: The positioning stand(Ch.2) is a multi-arm stand-alone system which occupies workspace adjacent to the surgical bed. This can be avoided by another design version consisting of single modular arms which can be attached to the bedside structure directly. These miniaturized arms with far less required space(due to their direct attachment to the bed-side instead of a separate column structure) can be used based on their desired configurations for the procedure by their attachment to the bedside. However to achieve this, the naturally balanced SCARA configuration of current design has to be compromised with some other possibly unbalanced arms design(Table 2.1).

II - Tendon Actuated Flexible Stem: The design of flexible stems with spherical joints can be further developed by implementing Servo-controls for actuation of tendons. However, the main challenge is to be able to control both the position as well as the tension force of the tendons. This is necessary since the joints movement is directly proportional to the movements of tendons , while their locking (based on the joints friction[App.A]) is directly proportional to the tension of tendons. The tendon-actuated flexible stems can have application not only as laparoscopic extenders, but also in other fields of applications such as manipulators for inspection and maintenance of nuclear facilities[92].

III - Miniaturized Force Reflecting Grasper: For practical use of the force reflecting grasper (Chapter 5) in laparoscopy, there exists a major challenge of miniaturization of the tunable spring and its actuation mechanism, which requires further research and developmental work. In order to make the tunable spring compact, one possible avenue is that, instead of leaf spring, other more compact types of spring such as curved or spiral springs can be used. However, the problem of actuation mechanism of the spring still remains. Another novel approach is possible by using compact hydraulic actuators at the handle instead of tunable springs, that can simulate the effects of the tunable spring. The small hydraulic cylinder can be actuated remotely through flexible tubes by a proportional pressure control valve and a hydraulic power unit.

IV - Hybrid haptic interface: The tunable spring is effective in reflecting large forces from the handle to the grasper of laparoscopic forceps, and vice versa, with low operational bandwidth($\leq 2Hz$, Chapter 5). This low-bandwidth haptic interface could be complemented by directing the higher frequency part of the sensed grasping force to piezo-electric actuators mounted in the handle of the grasper. This hybrid haptic interface is capable of reflecting both large forces (with low bandwidth) as well as small forces (with high bandwidth) for vibration and "jitter" sensing while manipulating hard objects. This type of hybrid haptic interface could have various applications in passive linkage-mechanisms(e.g. laparoscopic graspers) where the quality of force reflection over the whole range of bandwidth is hampered due to the presence of friction, backlash, or high inertia.

V - Tele-Operated Master-Slave system: The future of laparoscopy lies in tele-surgery, based on the robotic extenders suggested in Chapter 6, as the slave part with 6 DOF. Also by additional design work and prototyping of the master arm, it is possible to develop a complete tele-operated system for laparoscopic surgery. Further enhancement of such a system requires sensing of forces(both the grasping and manipulating forces of tissue by the slave arm) and reflecting them to the hand of surgeon through the master arm by implementing bilateral tele-operation system[92].

Appendix A
General Friction Models of Joints

In general, all linkage mechanisms and multi-body systems consist of joints and linkages, and rotary joints are the most commonly used type of joint in them. Rotary joints consist of two general categories: a) revolute joints (providing 1 DOF), and b) spherical joints (up to 3 DOF). The revolute pin joints and spherical socket-ball joints are used when the requirements include: a) relatively high radial loads at the joints, b) very high stiffness of the joints to reduce the vibrational tendencies of the system, and c) simple and compact joints. However, these two types of joints have disadvantages (compared to low friction bearings with intermediate rolling elements) such as: a) lower operational speed, b) relatively shorter service life, and c) higher friction. This higher level of friction forces us to estimate/predict the frictional moment caused by the joints more accurately both in statically and dynamic cases. The motivation for accurate modeling of frictional moments in these types of joints, is explained further by the following examples:

I) In the static cases (e.g. truss-cell systems[89], or endoscopic multi-jointed devices [81][32]), it is desired to predict/estimate the maximum frictional moment capacity of the staticly locked joints under different loading conditions.

II) In the dynamic cases of multi-body systems, the frictional moment at each joint is a contributing factor in the dynamic interaction between bodies. For accurate modeling of the system, it is essential to model frictional moment with the required accuracy[77][42][46].

III) Another specific example (as both static and dynamic cases) is the flexible stem in endoscopic tools which consists of several spherical joints (Fig.A.1). This allows the tool's tip to have two degrees of freedom inside the abdominal cavity. Each joint is actuated by tendon-like wires at the periphery. The unique feature of this design is that these joints are held together, moved, and locked by changing the tension in the tendons. In the static case, when the joints are locked, the tension in the wires should exceed some minimum limit in order to prevent the joints from any slipping while manipulating tissues and organs. However, in the dynamic case of moving joints, the tension must be reduced in some of the wires to allow the joints to rotate in the desired direction. In both of these cases it is important to estimate accurately the frictional moments of joints which are controlled by the tension of tendons.

As mentioned above, there are several papers related to experimental applications/studies of Coulomb frictional moment of joints [46][81][89], as well as general theoretical studies [42][77]. In all of these works, it is assumed that joints are absolutely rigid, and the contact is modeled as a point contact in the spherical socket-ball joints, and a line contact in revolute joints, where all the frictional force is concentrated. The

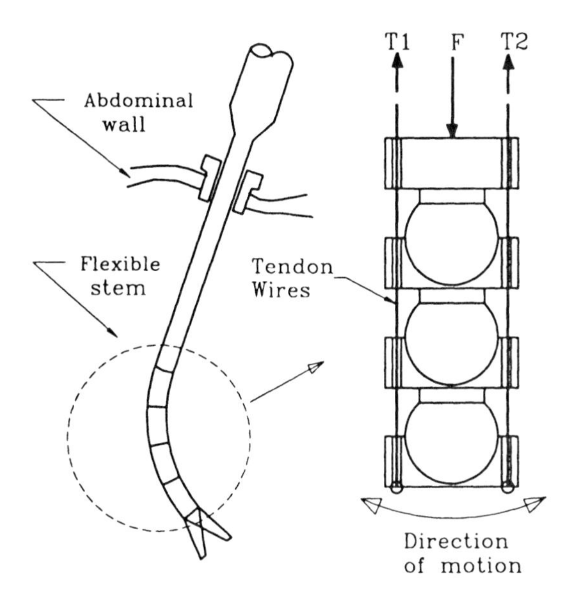

Figure A.1. The flexible stem of an endoscopic tool.

analysis has led to a simple mathematical model to predict the frictional moment.

In general there exist a contact area formed due to the elastic deformation of the joint where Coulomb friction is present. In this appendix, contacts in the joints are considered elastic and using the elliptic load distribution over the contact surfaces, new models are developed (Sec.2, and 3) which can predict/estimate the frictional moments with better accuracies (Sec.4, and 5). Finally, mathematical models for estimating the range of clearance in the joints, that ensures full contact and maximum stiffness of the pin and socket-ball joints, are presented (Sec.6).

1. PRELIMINARY ANALYSIS

The simple derivation of the current model is demonstrated here by the assumption of absolute rigidity of the joint with a point contact between its surfaces (Fig.A.2, the cross sectional view for both cases). The force F is the resultant external load acting on the joint (Fig.A.2), and the basic equilibrium of forces and moments for both cases are :

$$\sum F_x = -N \sin\theta_0 + \mu N \cos\theta_0 = 0$$
$$\sum F_y = N \cos\theta_0 + \mu N \sin\theta_0 = F$$
$$\sum M_o = \mu N R = Fl$$

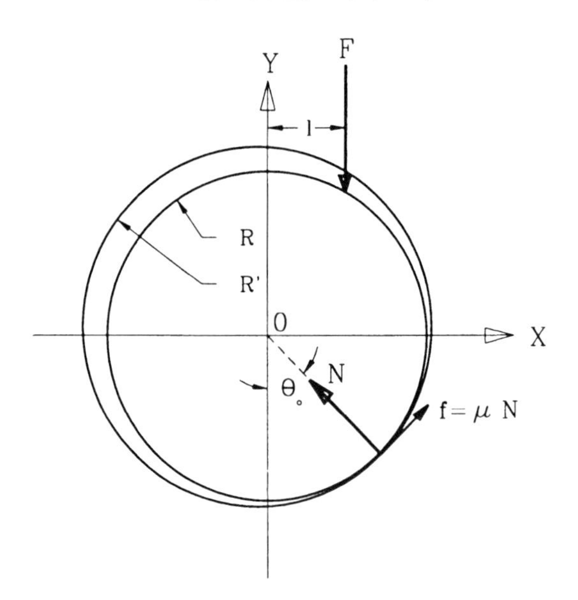

Figure A.2. The rigid joint under load F.

where: N = The reaction force at the contact point.
l = The distance of force F to the center of joint.
θ_0 = The equilibrium angle of contact point.
μ = The coefficient of friction between the two surfaces of joint.

The first equation leads to: $\tan\theta_0 = \mu$, and solving the other two equations, results $N = F/\sqrt{1+\mu^2}$, and :

$$\frac{l}{R} = \frac{\mu}{\sqrt{1+\mu^2}} \tag{A.1}$$

By using the above equations, the frictional moment acting on the joint ($M = \mu NR$) would be:

$$M = F \times R\frac{\mu}{\sqrt{1+\mu^2}} \tag{A.2}$$

and for small values of μ (e.g. $\mu < 0.3$), the value of $\sqrt{1+\mu^2}$ can be approximated to be equal to 1, and Eq.s (A.1) and (A.2) reduce to: $l/R = \mu$, and $M = \mu FR$.

Equation (A.2) is used extensively in the literature [42][46][77][81][89] to predict frictional moment in revolute or spherical joints. However, the above simplified analysis does not consider the elasticity of the joints. The following sections take into account the effects of the local elastic deformation in revolute pin joints, and spherical socket-ball joints, in order to estimate the Coulomb frictional moment more realistically, and with higher accuracy.

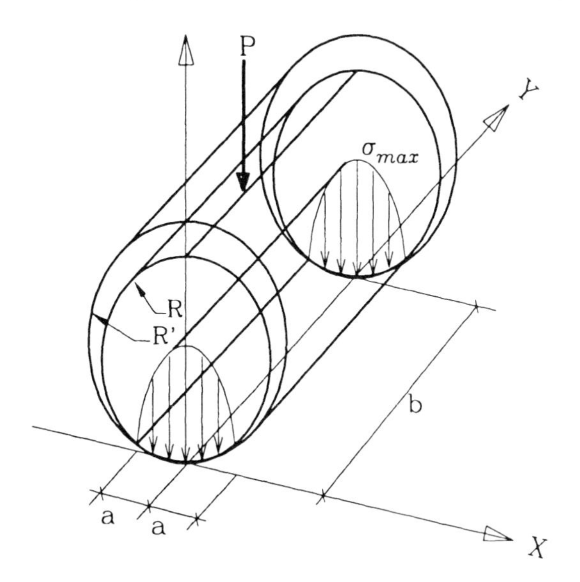

Figure A.3. The stress distribution between two cylindrical surfaces.

2. REVOLUTE PIN JOINTS

This section first presents the study of the stress distribution on the contact area of revolute joint, then by applying the Coulomb friction law at the contact area, the equilibrium analysis is carried out.

2.1 THE RADIAL STRESS DISTRIBUTION

The radial contact stress σ_r between the two cylindrical surfaces of radii R and R' due to the deformation is known[11][54] to have an elliptical distribution, or:

$$\sigma_r = \sigma_{max}\sqrt{1 - \frac{x^2}{a^2}} \tag{A.3}$$

When the material of the two surfaces are the same, with the module of elasticity E and Poisson ratio $\nu \approx 0.3$ (true for most alloys), the maximum radial stress σ_{max} at the center line of contact region is :

$$\sigma_{max} = 0.418\left[\frac{PE}{b}\left(\frac{R' - R}{RR'}\right)\right]^{1/2} \tag{A.4}$$

and the width of contact area ($= 2a$, Fig.A.3) can be obtained by :

$$a = R\sin\alpha = 1.52\left[\frac{P}{Eb}\frac{R'R}{R' - R}\right]^{1/2} \tag{A.5}$$

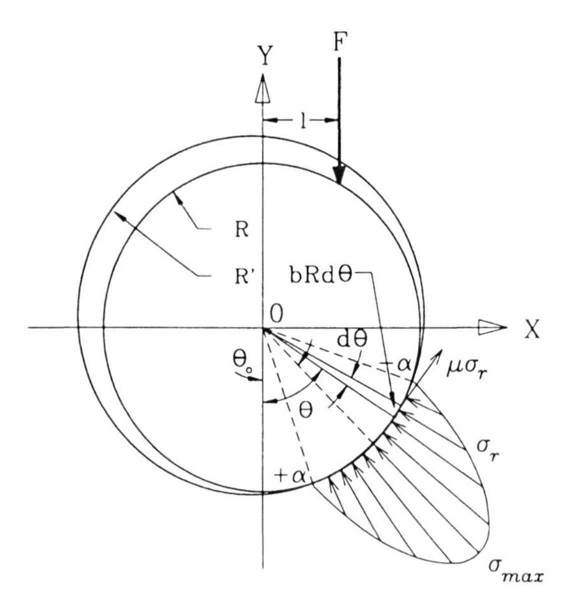

Figure A.4. The revolute pin joint under load F.

Where : b = The axial width of the revolute joint (Fig.A.3).
$P = F \cos\theta_0$ = The radial component of load F.
α = Half of the maximum angular contact between the two cylinders (Fig.A.4).

When the materials of the two surfaces are not the same, with different modules of elasticity E_1, E_2, and Poisson ratios ν_1, ν_2, then E in the above equation is replaced by $1.82E_1E_2/((1-\nu_2^2)E_1 + (1-\nu_1^2)E_2)$ [54].

Equation (A.3) is used for obtaining the radial stress distribution, and the Coulomb frictional law ($\sigma_t = \mu\sigma_r$) for obtaining the tangential stress distribution between two cylindrical surfaces of the joint.

2.2 EQUILIBRIUM ANALYSIS

Given the stress distributions on cylindrical surfaces, it is possible to write equilibrium equations of forces and moments. The components of forces acting on an infinitesimal area of contact $b.R.d\theta$ (Fig.A.4) are:

$$\sum \mathbf{d\vec{F}} = \sigma_r.b.R.d\theta[(\mu\cos\theta - \sin\theta)\hat{\mathbf{i}} + (\cos\theta + \mu\sin\theta)\hat{\mathbf{j}}] \qquad \text{(A.6)}$$

Where $\sigma_r = \sigma_{max}\sqrt{1 - \frac{R^2}{a^2}\sin^2(\theta - \theta_0)}$ is obtained from Eq.(A.3).

By integrating over the contact area, equilibrium equations of forces along x, y, and moment around z axis (Fig.A.4) could be written as:

$$\sum \mathbf{F}_x = \int_{\theta_0-\alpha}^{\theta_0+\alpha} \sum \mathbf{d\vec{F}}.\hat{\mathbf{i}} =$$

$$\int_{\theta_0-\alpha}^{\theta_0+\alpha} bR\sigma_{max}(\mu\cos\theta - \sin\theta)\sqrt{1-\frac{R^2}{a^2}\sin^2(\theta-\theta_0)}.d\theta = 0 \quad \text{(A.7)}$$

$$\sum \mathbf{F}_y = \int_{\theta_0-\alpha}^{\theta_0+\alpha} \sum \mathbf{d\vec{F}}.\hat{\mathbf{j}} =$$

$$\int_{\theta_0-\alpha}^{\theta_0+\alpha} bR\sigma_{max}(\mu\sin\theta + \cos\theta)\sqrt{1-\frac{R^2}{a^2}\sin^2(\theta-\theta_0)}.d\theta = F \quad \text{(A.8)}$$

$$\sum \mathbf{M}_o = \int_{\theta_0-\alpha}^{\theta_0+\alpha} \left[\vec{\mathbf{R}} \times \sum \mathbf{d\vec{F}}\right].\hat{\mathbf{k}} =$$

$$\int_{\theta_0-\alpha}^{\theta_0+\alpha} \mu bR^2\sigma_{max}\sqrt{1-\frac{R^2}{a^2}\sin^2(\theta-\theta_0)}.d\theta = F.l \quad \text{(A.9)}$$

Where: θ_0= the angle where maximum radial stress occurs (Fig.A.4).
$\vec{\mathbf{R}} = R(\sin\theta\hat{\mathbf{i}} - \cos\theta\hat{\mathbf{j}})$
l = the distance between force F and y axis (Fig.A.4).

By substituting for $a = R\sin\alpha$, $u = \theta - \theta_0$, and the trigonometric expansion of Eq.(A.7) and (A.8), they can be solved and provide the following equations:

$$\tan\theta_0 = \mu \quad \text{(A.10)}$$

$$F = \frac{\pi b.R}{2}\sigma_{max}(1+\mu^2)^{1/2}\sin\alpha \quad \text{(A.11)}$$

On the other hand, Eq.(A.9) can not be solved analytically since it is an elliptic integral. There are various approaches of finding the solution for (A.9).

I) Numerical Integration : This method could be applied by using numerical integration algorithms to each individual case, however it is computationally intensive, and time consuming. This is specially true when the solution is needed for dynamic cases (such as the endoscopic flexible extenders), where load and other parameters are constantly changing.

II) Tabulated Values : There are tables for different kinds of elliptic integrals that could be used[12] to solve Eq.(A.9). Although not practical, they are used in this appendix (Table.A.1) to verify the results of next method (*Expansion Series*), and based on that, develop a closed-form approximate solution.

III) Expansion Series : Approximation is possible by obtaining series expansion of Eq.(A.9). For this purpose first let $K = R/a$ and $u = \theta - \theta_0$ to get Eq.(A.9) in the following form:

$$\frac{Fl}{\mu b R^2 \sigma_{max}} = \int_{-\alpha}^{\alpha} \sqrt{1 - K^2 \sin u^2} du = 2\mathcal{E}(\alpha, K) \quad \text{(A.12)}$$

Where $\mathcal{E}(\alpha, K)$ is defined as *the normal elliptic integral of the second kind*[12], that could be represented with expansion series if $K < 1$. However in our case $K \geq 1$ since: $K = R/a$, and $a = R \sin \alpha$, so $K = 1/\sin \alpha$, since $1 \geq \sin \alpha \geq 0$ which results in: $K \geq 1$. Therefore, it is necessary to use *Reciprocal Modulus Transformation*[12] of $\mathcal{E}(\alpha, K)$ as:

$\mathcal{E}(\alpha, K) = [\mathcal{E}(\beta, k) - (1 - k^2)\mathcal{F}(\beta, k)]/k$

Where $k = 1/K = \sin \alpha$, and $\beta = \sin^{-1}(K \sin \alpha) = \sin^{-1}(1) = \pi/2$. Also $\mathcal{F}(\beta, k)$ is *the normal elliptic integral of the first kind.* Then equation (A.12) is transformed to:

$$\frac{Fl}{\mu b R^2 \sigma_{max}} = 2\mathcal{E}(\alpha, K) = 2[\mathcal{E}(\pi/2, k) - (1 - k^2)\mathcal{F}(\pi/2, k)]/k \quad \text{(A.13)}$$

Now by substituting (11) in (13), it further reduces to:

$$\frac{l}{R} = \frac{4\mathcal{E}(\alpha, K)}{\pi \sin \alpha} \frac{\mu}{\sqrt{1 + \mu^2}} = C_\alpha \frac{\mu}{\sqrt{1 + \mu^2}} \quad \text{(A.14)}$$

Where

$$C_\alpha = \frac{4\mathcal{E}(\alpha, K)}{\pi \sin \alpha} = \frac{4}{\pi}[\mathcal{E}(\pi/2, k) - (1 - k^2)\mathcal{F}(\pi/2, k)]/k^2 \quad \text{(A.15)}$$

The expansion series of $\mathcal{E}$, and $\mathcal{F}$[12] can be used to obtain an expansion series for C_α by applying them to Eq.(A.15) as the followings:

$\mathcal{E}(\pi/2, k) = \frac{\pi}{2}\left[1 - \frac{1}{4}k^2 - \frac{3}{64}k^4 - \frac{5}{256}k^6 - \frac{175}{16384}k^8 - .....\right]$

$\mathcal{F}(\pi/2, k) = \frac{\pi}{2}\left[1 + \frac{1}{4}k^2 + \frac{9}{64}k^4 + \frac{25}{256}k^6 + \frac{1225}{16384}k^8 + ...\right]$

$$C_\alpha = 1 + \frac{1}{8}k^2 + \frac{3}{64}k^4 + \frac{25}{1024}k^6 + \frac{245}{16384}k^8 + ... \quad \text{(A.16)}$$

On the other hand, the tabulated values of $\mathcal{E}$ and $\mathcal{F}$[12] are used, and the following values of C_α based on Eq.(A.16) are calculated (Table.A.1) and plotted versus α in Fig.A.5 (shown by small circles).

Comparing the results of these two approaches shows that, the series (A.16) converges to the final values of C_α (Table.A.1) very slowly as the

Table A.1. The values of C_α for different contact angles α .

α	$k = \sin\alpha$	$\mathcal{E}(\pi/2, k)$	$\mathcal{F}(\pi/2, k)$	$2\mathcal{E}(\alpha, K)$	C_α
0	0.000	1.57080	1.570796	0.0000	1.000
5	0.087	1.567809	1.573792	0.1370	1.001
15	0.259	1.544150	1.598142	0.4100	1.008
30	0.500	1.467462	1.685750	0.8126	1.035
45	0.707	1.350644	1.854075	1.1981	1.079
60	0.866	1.211056	2.156516	1.5517	1.141
75	0.966	1.076405	2.768063	1.8448	1.216
90	1.000	1.000000	∞	2.0000	1.273

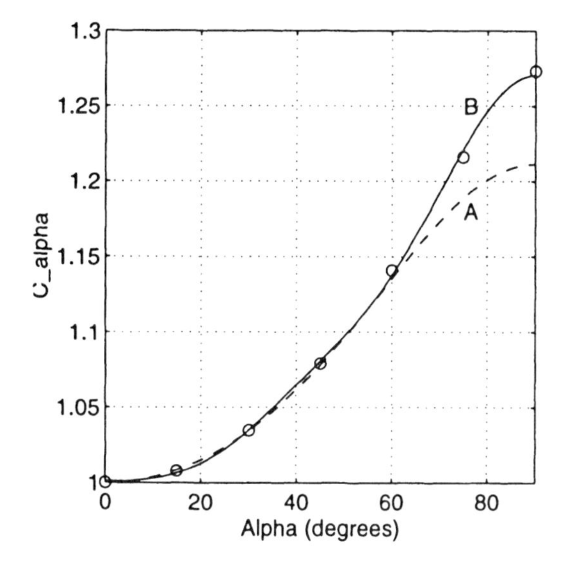

Figure A.5. C_α vs. α for revolute pin joints.

number of elements in the series are increased. For example, even the summation of the first five elements of the series results in 5% deviation for large values of α (shown by the dashed line A, in Fig.A.5) from the tabulated values.

IV) Curve Fitting : By curve fitting techniques (to the data points of C_α from Table.A.1), it is possible to obtain functions with better accuracy compared to the results of expansion series with limited number of elements. For example, by knowing the type of polynomial obtained from the series (i.e. Eq.A.16), the function $C_\alpha = 1 + Ak^2 + Bk^4 + Ck6 + Dk^8$ could be solved by least square method for the tabulated values of

C_α (from Table.A.1), to obtain the coefficients: A, B, C, and D. This results in:

$$C_\alpha = 1 + 0.0477k^2 + 0.5744k^4 - 1.051k^6 + 0.6982k^8 \tag{A.17}$$

The above equation has less than 1% deviation from the values of C_α over the whole range of α (shown by the solid line B, in Fig.A.5). This is a reasonable level of accuracy for most practical applications, but other optimal curve fitting techniques might even achieve higher accuracies.

Now by having the equation of C_α, the final frictional moment of the revolute pin joint can be written as :

$$M = F \times l =$$

$$F \times R(1+0.0477\sin^2\alpha+0.5744\sin^4\alpha-1.051\sin^6\alpha+0.6982\sin^8\alpha)\frac{\mu}{\sqrt{1+\mu^2}} \tag{A.18}$$

Where α can be obtained from (A.5) and (A.10) as:

$$\alpha = \sin^{-1}\left[\left(\frac{2.31F}{Eb\sqrt{1+\mu^2}}.\frac{R'/R}{R'-R}\right)^{1/2}\right].$$

From the above equation it is evident that the value of M for some specific force F depends only on the parameter l. So the ratio l/R $(= M/FR)$ can be considered as a dimensionless index that represents the maximum moment capacity of the joint, regardless of the revolute joints dimensions.

l/R from equation (A.14) is plotted for different values of μ and α in Fig.A.6. In this plot, the curve corresponding to $\alpha = 0$ represents rigid joint model (since, for $\alpha = 0 : C_\alpha = 1$, and Eq.A.14 converts to Eq.A.1), and comparing it to the full contact case (where $\alpha = 90°$), Eq.(A.1) has a deviation of 21% from Eq.(A.18). This could result in the same amount of error, if Eq.(A.1) is used for a full contact case. Actually, the straight line approximation $l/R = \mu$ provides much better approximation for near full contact conditions than its parent equation (A.1). However, there is no need for approximation anymore, the new model (A.18) provides accurate estimation of M for any condition of friction and contact angle.

3. SPHERICAL SOCKET-BALL JOINTS

In this section, almost same procedure as Sec.2 is applied to spherical socket-ball joints. First, the stress distribution on the contact area of the spherical joint is studied, then by applying Coulomb friction law at the contact area the equilibrium analysis is carried out.

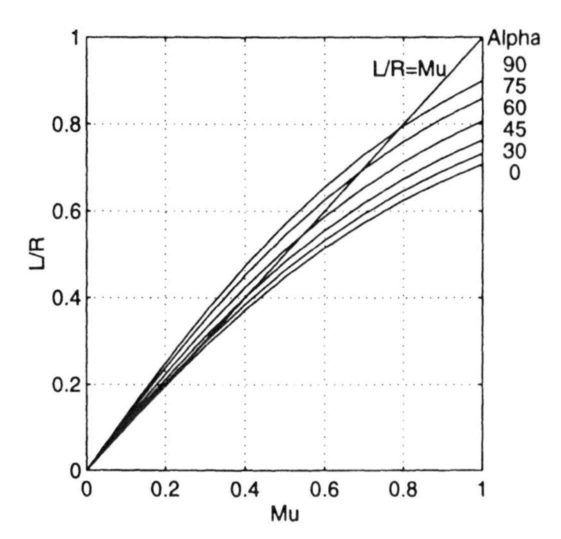

Figure A.6. l/R vs. μ for revolute pin joints.

3.1 THE RADIAL STRESS DISTRIBUTION

Similar to the cylindrical case (Eq.A3), the radial contact stress σ_r between the two spherical surfaces of radii R and R' due to deformation are known[11][54] to be an elliptical distribution as well. However, the elliptic distribution is along two axes (i.e. X, and Y axis, Fig.A.7) :

$$\sigma_r = \sigma_{max}\sqrt{1 - \frac{x^2}{a^2} - \frac{y^2}{a^2}} \qquad (A.19)$$

When the material of the two surfaces are the same, with the module of elasticity E and Poisson ratio $\nu \approx 0.3$ (true for most alloys), the maximum radial stress σ_{max} at the center of contact region is :

$$\sigma_{max} = 0.389[PE^2(\frac{R - R'}{RR'})^2]^{1/3} \qquad (A.20)$$

And the radius of contact region ($= a$, Fig.A.7) can be obtained by :

$$a = R\sin\alpha = 1.11[\frac{P}{E}\frac{RR'}{R - R'}]^{1/3} \qquad (A.21)$$

Where : $P = F\cos\theta_0$ = The radial component of F.
α = Half of the maximum contact angle between the two spheres.

However, if the materials of the two surfaces are not the same, then E in the above equation has to be changed with $1.82E_1E_2/((1 - \nu_2^2)E_1 + (1 - \nu_1^2)E_2)$ as described in Sec.A.2.

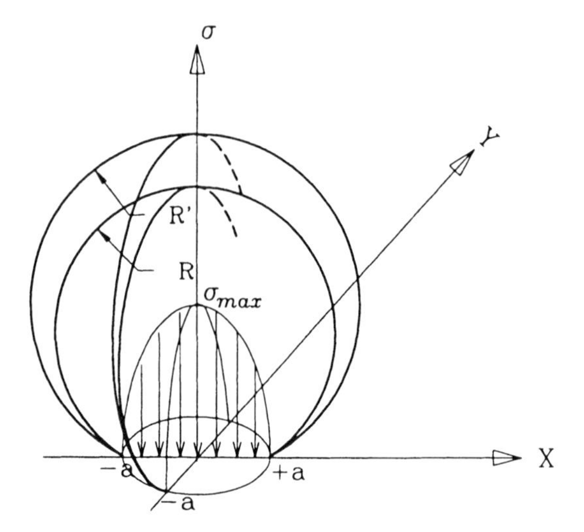

Figure A.7. The stress distribution between two spherical surfaces.

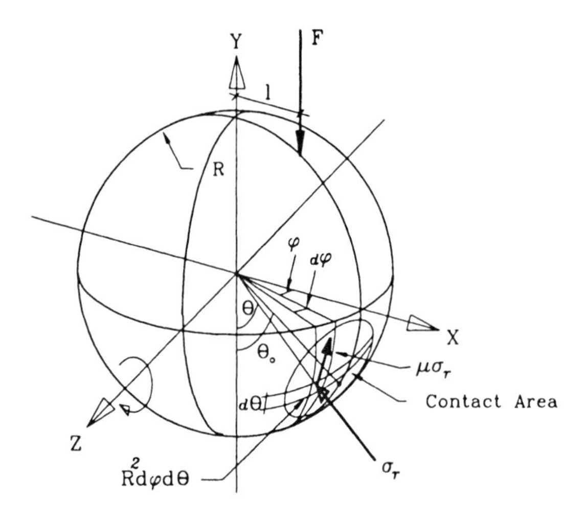

Figure A.8. The spherical socket ball joint under load F.

3.2 EQUILIBRIUM ANALYSIS

Based on the stress distribution on the spherical surface, the equilibrium equations of forces and moments can be obtained. First, by considering forces acting on an infinitesimal area, then integrating it over the whole contact area. The components of forces (normal and frictional tangent forces) acting on an infinitesimal area of contact $R^2 d\phi d\theta$ (Fig.A.8) are:

$$\sum d\vec{\mathbf{F}} =$$

$$\sigma_r.R^2\left[(-\cos\phi\sin\theta\hat{\mathbf{i}}+\cos\theta\cos\phi\hat{\mathbf{j}}-\sin\phi\hat{\mathbf{k}})+\mu(\sin\theta\hat{\mathbf{j}}+\cos\theta\hat{\mathbf{i}})\right]d\phi d\theta \tag{A.22}$$

By integrating over the contact area, equilibrium equations of forces along x, y, and moment around z axis (Fig.A.8) could be written as:

$$\sum\vec{\mathbf{F}}_x=\int_{\theta_0-\alpha}^{\theta_0+\alpha}\int_{-\alpha'}^{+\alpha'}\sum d\vec{\mathbf{F}}.\hat{\mathbf{i}}=\int_{\theta_0-\alpha}^{\theta_0+\alpha}\int_{-\alpha'}^{+\alpha'}R^2\sigma_r(\mu\cos\theta-\cos\phi\sin\theta)d\phi d\theta=0 \tag{A.23}$$

$$\sum\vec{\mathbf{F}}_y=\int_{\theta_0-\alpha}^{\theta_0+\alpha}\int_{-\alpha'}^{+\alpha'}\sum d\vec{\mathbf{F}}.\hat{\mathbf{j}}=\int_{\theta_0-\alpha}^{\theta_0+\alpha}\int_{-\alpha'}^{+\alpha'}R^2\sigma_r(\cos\theta\cos\phi+\mu\sin\theta)d\phi d\theta=F \tag{A.24}$$

$$\sum\vec{\mathbf{M}}_z=\int_{\theta_0-\alpha}^{\theta_0+\alpha}\int_{-\alpha'}^{+\alpha'}\left[\vec{\mathbf{R}}\times\sum d\vec{\mathbf{F}}\right].\hat{\mathbf{k}}=\int_{\theta_0-\alpha}^{\theta_0+\alpha}\int_{-\alpha'}^{+\alpha'}\mu R^2\sigma_r\cos\phi d\phi d\theta=F.l \tag{A.25}$$

Where, $\sigma_r=\sigma_{max}\sqrt{1-[\frac{R}{a}\sin(\theta-\theta_0)]^2-[\frac{R}{a}\sin\phi]^2}$
$\vec{\mathbf{R}}=R(\cos\phi\sin\theta\hat{\mathbf{i}}-\cos\phi\cos\theta\hat{\mathbf{j}}+\sin\phi\hat{\mathbf{k}})$
l = the distance between force F and y axis (Fig.A.8).
θ_0 = The angular position of center of the contact area (Fig.A.8).
$\alpha'=\sin^{-1}\sqrt{\sin^2\alpha-\sin^2(\theta-\theta_0)}$

After expansion of Eq.(23) and (24), they convert into elliptic integral forms which do not have analytical solutions. However, it is possible numerically to verify that the Eq.(A.23) leads to the same equation: $\tan\theta_0=\mu$, for different values of μ and α. Now, by knowing $\theta_0=\tan^{-1}\mu$, it is possible to find the radial component of force F (i.e. $P=F\cos\theta_0$), which drives the two spherical surfaces into each other radially, and is the same as force P in Eq.(20) and (21). As a result we can have:
$P=F\cos\theta_0=F/\sqrt{1+\mu^2}$

On the other hand, by multiplying Eq.(A.20) by square of Eq.(A.21), it is possible to obtain a relation between σ_{max} and P as :
$\sigma_{max}(R\sin\alpha)^2=0.388(1.11)^2\left[P^3(\frac{E.\Delta R.R}{E.R.\Delta R})^2\right]^{1/3}=0.388(1.11)^2P$

Replacing $P=F/\sqrt{1+\mu^2}$ in the above equation, a relationship between F, and σ_{max} can be obtained without solving Eq.(A.24) as followings :

$$\sigma_{max}=\frac{0.388(1.11)^2}{R^2\sin^2\alpha\sqrt{1+\mu^2}}F \tag{A.26}$$

Now by substituting σ_{max} (A.26) in the trigonometric form of equation (A.19):

$$\sigma_r=\sigma_{max}\sqrt{1-[\frac{R}{a}\sin(\theta-\theta_0)]^2-[\frac{R}{a}\sin\phi]^2}=$$

$$\frac{0.388(1.11)^2}{R^2\sin^2\alpha\sqrt{1+\mu^2}}F\sqrt{1-[\frac{R}{a}\sin(\theta-\theta_0)]^2-[\frac{R}{a}\sin\phi]^2}$$

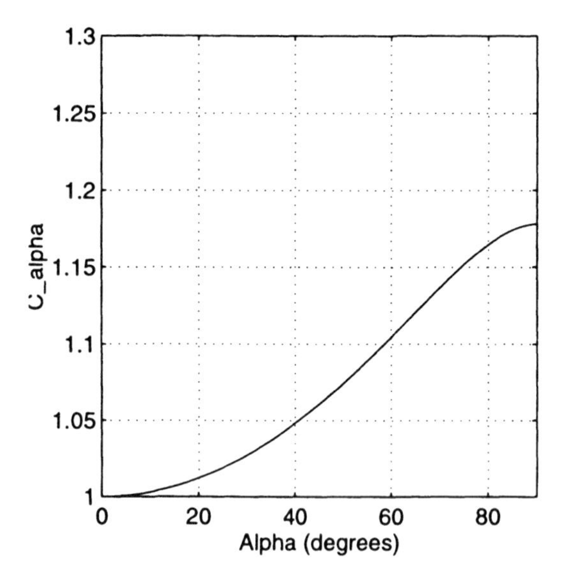

Figure A.9. C_α vs. α for spherical socket ball joints.

provides us with σ_r, which can be used in Eq.(A.25). This makes it possible to integrate Eq.(A.25), and obtain:

$$\pi\mu\frac{0.388(1.11)^2}{R^2\sin^2\alpha\sqrt{1+\mu^2}}FR^3\left[\cos\alpha-\alpha\frac{\cos 2\alpha}{\sin\alpha}\right]=Fl$$

after simplification it leads to:

$$\frac{l}{R}=0.75\left[\frac{\cos\alpha}{\sin^2\alpha}-\alpha\frac{\cos 2\alpha}{\sin^3\alpha}\right]\frac{\mu}{\sqrt{1+\mu^2}} \tag{A.27}$$

This equation (A.27) has the same basic structure as Eq.(A.14) in the case of revolute pin joint (i.e. $l/R=C_\alpha\mu/\sqrt{1+\mu^2}$). However, C_α in this case is:

$$C_\alpha=0.75\left[\frac{\cos\alpha}{\sin^2\alpha}-\alpha\frac{\cos 2\alpha}{\sin^3\alpha}\right] \tag{A.28}$$

C_α is plotted versus α in Fig.A.9, that can be interpreted as the deviation of elastic joint (as a more realistic assumption), compared to the absolute rigid joint (as an ideal case, where $C_\alpha=1$).

Now, by using Eq.(A.28), the frictional moment of the spherical joint would be:

$$M=F\times l=\frac{3F\times R}{4}\left[\frac{\cos\alpha}{\sin^2\alpha}-\alpha\frac{\cos 2\alpha}{\sin^3\alpha}\right]\frac{\mu}{\sqrt{1+\mu^2}} \tag{A.29}$$

Where, α can be obtained from (A.21) as: $\alpha=\sin^{-1}\left[\left(\frac{1.367F}{ER\Delta R\sqrt{1+\mu^2}}\right)^{1/3}\right]$

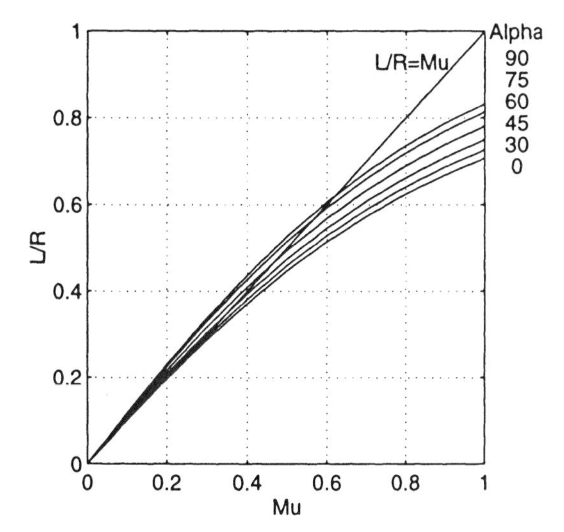

Figure A.10. l/R vs. μ for spherical socket ball joints.

Same as previous section (Sec.A.2), l/R is the dimensionless parameter that represents the frictional moment capacity (M), of the spherical socket ball joint regardless of its size. Hence, l/R of Eq.(A.27) is plotted for different values of μ and α as shown in Fig.A.10. In this plot, the curve corresponding to $\alpha = 0$, represents the rigid joint model, and comparing to full contact case (where $\alpha = 90°$), Eq.(A.1) has a deviation of about 15%. This means, Eq.(A.1) would result in 15% error, if used when the joint is in full contact.

4. DISCUSSION I: CONTACT ANGLES AND LOADS

Based on the previous analysis, we have presented the mathematical models (Eq.s A.18, and A.29) that can predict the frictional moment M of the joints as a function of the contact angle α, and μ. However, to apply these models effectively, it is important to know, under what range of loads on the joint, the value of α (and subsequently C_α, and M) is affected mostly. To clarify this in more detail, the following questions must be addressed and discussed:

I) In what minimal range of loads does the joint still behaves as a rigid joint (i.e. $\alpha \approx 0$, and $C_\alpha \approx 1$)?

II) In what intermediate range of loads does the joint have partial contact as would an elastic joint (i.e. $0 < \alpha < 90°$)?

III) In what maximal range of loads does the joint have full contact as would an elastic joint (i.e. $\alpha = 90°$)?

In order to answer the above questions, first we have to find the maximum load capacity of the joint P_{max}, as an upper bound limit, as well as a relative scale of comparison for other smaller loads (as the ratio P/P_{max}). The reason that P has been used here instead of the load force F is that the radial load $P(= F\cos\theta_0)$ is the only contributing component of load F which is used in the computation of σ_{max} in Eq.s (A.4) and (A.20).

Let us first consider the revolute pin joints. Based on the strength of material (as the design criteria for maximum loading of joints), the maximum radial force P_{max} that can be exerted on the joint must not induce larger stresses than the allowable stress $\frac{\sigma_y}{S}$, where σ_y is the yield stress of the joint's material and S is the safety factor of the design. Therefore σ_{max} in Eq.(A.4) can be replaced by $\frac{\sigma_y}{S}$ in order to find the maximum value of P defined as P_{max}:

$$P_{max} = \frac{5.72bRR'\sigma_y^2}{E\Delta RS^2} \approx \frac{5.72b(R\sigma_y)^2}{E\Delta RS^2} \tag{A.30}$$

Where $\Delta R = R' - R$.

On the other hand, the full contact between the two cylindrical surfaces of the joint happens when the contact angle is 180° (i.e. $\alpha = 90°$, Fig.A.4). Here, $P_{f.c.}$ is defined as the minimum radial force required to cause *full contact* in the joint (i.e. $\alpha = 90°$). A relation for $P_{f.c.}$ can be reached by substituting $\alpha = 90°$ in Eq.(A.5):

$a = R\sin(90°) = 1.52[\frac{P_{f.c.}}{Eb}\frac{RR'}{\Delta R}]^{1/2}$ And by assuming $R' \simeq R$, $P_{f.c.}$ would be:

$$P_{f.c.} \geq \frac{Eb\Delta R}{2.31} \tag{A.31}$$

Now by dividing (A.31) by (A.30), for revolute pin joints the ratio of $P_{f.c.}$ and P_{max} can be obtained as :

$$1 \geq \frac{P_{f.c.}}{P_{max}} \geq 0.076 \left[S\frac{\Delta R}{R}\frac{E}{\sigma_y}\right]^2 \tag{A.32}$$

Same can be done for spherical socket-ball joints, that yields the following:

$$1 \geq \frac{P_{f.c.}}{P_{max}} \geq 0.043 \left[S\frac{\Delta R}{R}\frac{E}{\sigma_y}\right]^3 \tag{A.33}$$

Table A.2. The typical calculated values of C_α, α, and $\frac{P}{P_{max}}$.

Type	Revolute Pin Joint			Spherical Socket-Ball Joint		
Contact	Low	partial	Full	Low	partial	Full
C_α	1.0 - 1.01	1.01 - 1.27	1.273	1.0 - 1.01	1.01 - 1.17	1.178
α	0 - 20	21 - 89	90	0 - 18	19 - 89	90
$\frac{P}{P_{max}}$	0 - 0.01	0.01 - 0.08	0.08 - 1.0	0 - 0.001	0.001 - 0.05	0.05 - 1.0

As an example, let us look at a steel joint with normal design parameters such as: $\sigma_y = 500MPa, E = 210GPa, R = 10mm, \Delta R = 0.01mm$, and the design safety factor of S=2.5 . Table.A.2 shows the typical calculated values for α, C_α, and $\frac{P}{P_{max}}$ for the revolute and spherical cases. In this table, low contact refers to the narrow range of α that corresponds to the range of $1 \leq C_\alpha \leq 1.01$. In other words, the low contact range represents the range of α (and the corresponding values of P/P_{max}), that $C_\alpha \simeq 1$, and the joint is still behaving rigidly under the very light load. The partial contact is defined as the range for which contact angle α is more than low contact range, but less than full contact ($\alpha = 90°$).

For revolute pin joints, from the above example it is apparent that, in order for the assumption of rigid joint to be accurate ($C_\alpha \simeq 1$) then P should not exceed 1% (and 0.1%, in the case of spherical joint) of the maximum allowable load P_{max}.

On the other hand, in the full contact columns, when the load P exceeds 8% and 5% of P_{max}, then C_α is equal to 1.273, and 1.178 for revolute and spherical joints respectively. This is more than 90% of the range of allowable load P_{max}. Therefore assuming $C_\alpha = 1.273$ (for revolute pin joints) and 1.178 (for spherical socket-ball) in the case of unknown loads (or when P is generally larger than $5-8\%$ of P_{max}), will result in a more accurate model than using the conventional model (where $C_\alpha = 1$, Eq.A.2).

5. DISCUSSION II: JOINTS CLEARANCE FOR MAXIMUM STIFFNESS

In the design of pin joints or socket-ball joints, the clearance is usually determined by the maximum allowable backlash play, or the tolerance of the manufacturing process, based on one of the running-fit standards of tolerance (e.g. ANSI B4.2). This might be sufficient for quasi-static applications where the rigidity of the joint is not a primary requirement. However for dynamic cases, or when vibratory loads are present, the

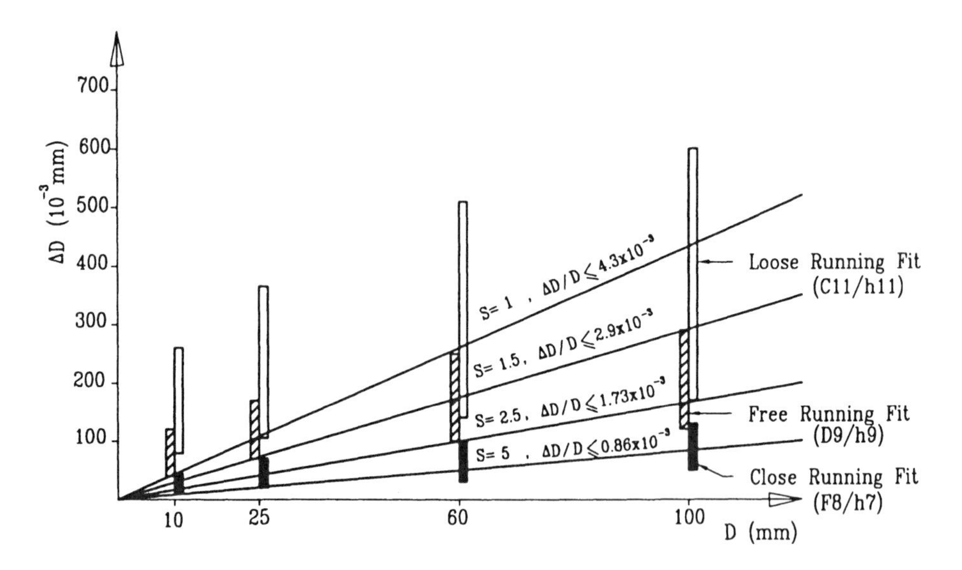

Figure A.11. Clearance in revolute pin joints for full contact.

high stiffness and rigidity of joints have the utmost importance. In this regard, the contact angle and joints clearance are discussed here to maximize joints stiffness (which is one of the main reasons for selection of pin or socket-ball joints compared to other bearings' designs, Sec.A.1).

The effect of contact angle on the stiffness of a socket-ball joint can be demonstrated by partial differentiation of the known equation of radial deformation of two spherical surfaces (of the same material): $\delta^3 = \frac{0.92P^2\Delta R}{ER^2}$[6]. Also substituting $P = \frac{a^3 E\Delta R}{1.36R^2}$ results for the stiffness :

$\frac{dP}{d\delta} = 1.4Ea$, where a is the contact length.

The above equation shows that the joint has no stiffness when $a \approx 0$, and to maximize its stiffness, the contact length, a, or angle α has to be maximized. Same type of equations can be developed for pin joints, which motivates us to develop equations for *the range of clearance* that *ensure full contact* under normal load conditions. This can be achieved by substituting $P_{f.c.} = P_{max}$ as the worst case which yields the largest $\frac{\Delta R}{R}$ in Eq.s (A.32), and (A.33), which after simplifications provides:

For revolute pin joints:

$$\frac{\Delta D}{D} = \frac{\Delta R}{R} \leq \frac{3.63\sigma_y}{S.E} \tag{A.34}$$

For socket-ball joints:

$$\frac{\Delta D}{D} = \frac{\Delta R}{R} \leq \frac{2.85\sigma_y}{S.E} \tag{A.35}$$

For instance, ΔD is plotted vs. D in Fig.A.11 based on Eq.(A.34), for a pin joint made of steel ($\sigma_y = 250MPa$, and $E = 210GPa$) with different safety factors ($S = 1$ to 5). This is compared with the design standards (ANSI B4.2-1978) for running fits (i.e. loose $C11/h11$, free $D9/h9$, and close running fits $F8/h7$).

Similar plots to Fig.A.11 (based on Eq.s A.34, and A.35) can help the designer as a new tool to improve the stiffness of the joints by choosing proper clearance for the load with the design safety factor (S), which provides full contact. For example, for a steel pin joint with diameter $D = 60mm$, and safety factor of $S = 2.5$, based on Fig.A.11, only close fit (i.e. $F8/h7$) or tighter fit ($\Delta D \leq 0.1mm$) can provide the condition of full contact.

6. SUMMARY

The elastic property of joints has led this study to the general formulation of the Coulomb frictional moment in the revolute pin joints or socket-ball joints as:

$$M = C_\alpha \frac{F \times R \times \mu}{\sqrt{1+\mu^2}}$$

Where the value of C_α can generally be determined in the following three cases:

Case 1: For low contact angles (e.g. $\alpha \leq 20°$), then $C_\alpha \simeq 1$. This corresponds to very light loads (e.g. about or less than 1% of joints allowable loads, Table.A.2), that the joint still acts as a rigid body.

Case 2: For partial contact (e.g. $20° < \alpha < 90°$) C_α can be calculated by the closed form equations (17), and (28) for the two cases.

Case 3: For full contact (that $\alpha = 90°$) C_α is equal to 1.273 ($= 4/\pi$), and 1.178 ($= 3\pi/8$) for the revolute and spherical joints respectively.

Case 3 is the dominant case of joints operation (more than 90% of the designed load range), that could be used for general estimations when the exact magnitude of load P, or contact angle α are unknown, but the loads are high enough to cause full contact or near full contact (e.g. $\frac{P}{P_{max}} > 0.08$, Table.A.2).

In comparison to the conventional friction model (where $C_\alpha = 1$), the new model with the value of C_α obtained according to case 2 or 3 can prevent up to 21% and 15% error in the Coulomb frictional moment estimation of pin and socket-ball joints respectively. This higher accuracy is specially important for better control, and dynamic modeling of multi-body systems with several joints in series (with the effect of cumulative error). One such case is the estimation of the frictional moments in the laparoscopic flexible stems for locking and motion control of the extenders.

Finally, to obtain maximum stiffness in the joints, the newly developed models for clearance (Eq.A.34, and A.35) can provide the designer with the proper range of clearance for both cases of revolute pin and socket-ball joints.

Appendix B
Sample Drawings of Flexible Stem

The drawings of following flexible stem designs of joints and grasper is included in this appendix as follows:

1. The single revolute joint design actuated by 4 bar linkages; Fig. B.1.
2. The multi-revolute joint design actuated by lead screws; Fig. B.2.
3. The multi-spherical joint design actuated by tendon wires; Fig. B.3.
4. The design of the grasper head actuated by a flexible shaft; Fig. B.4.

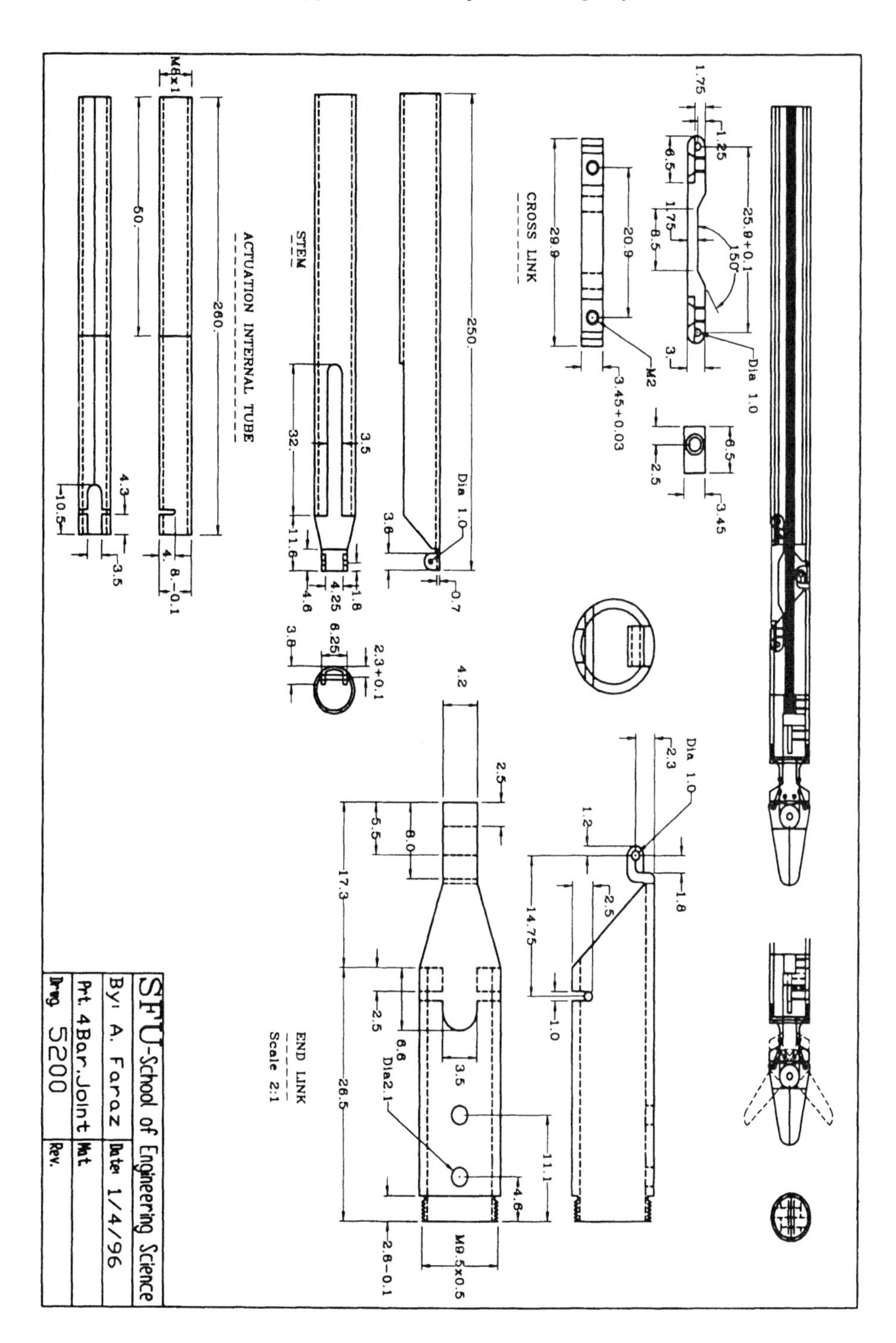

Figure B.1. The single revolute joint design actuated by 4 bar linkages.

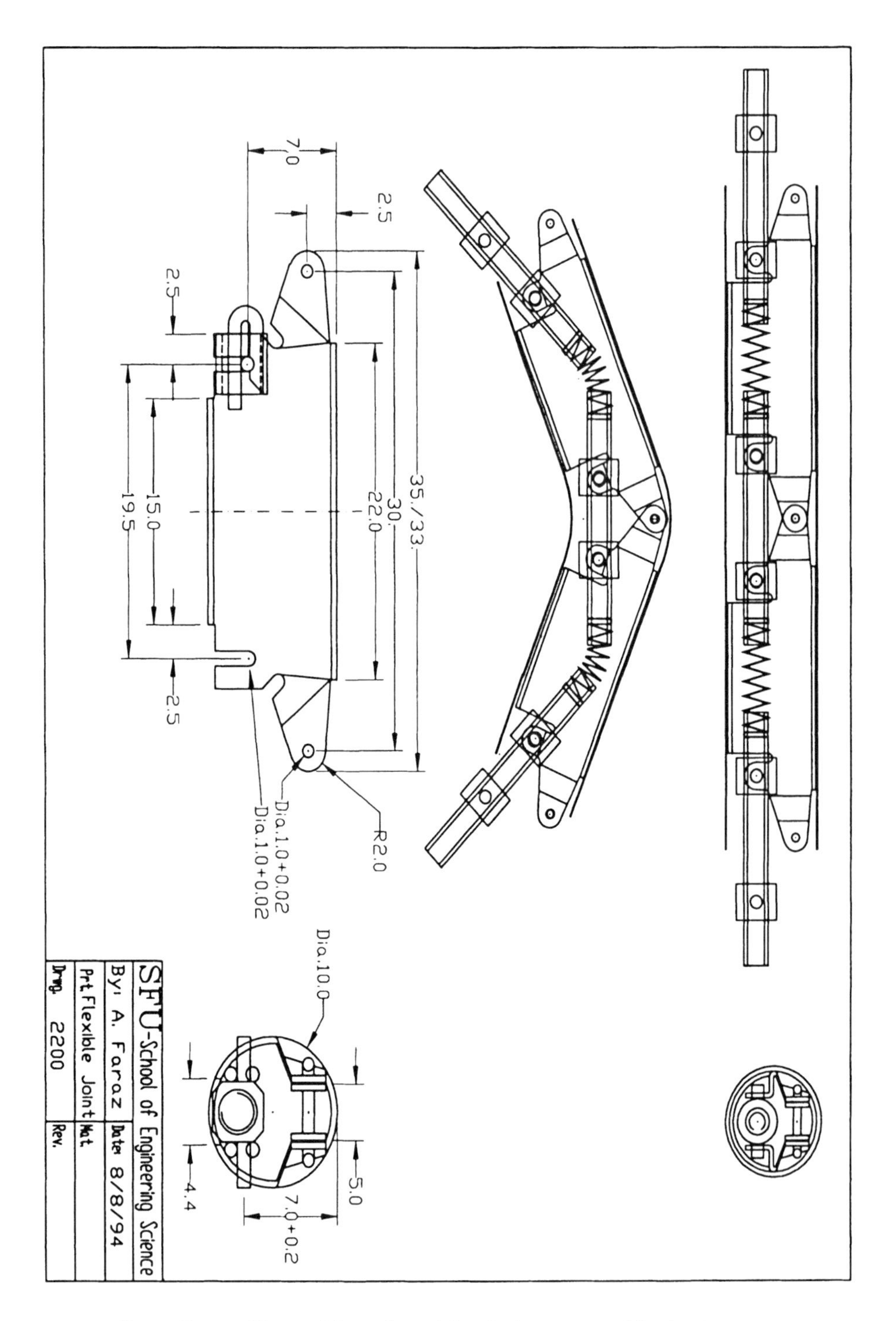

Figure B.2. The multi-revolute joint design actuated by lead screws.

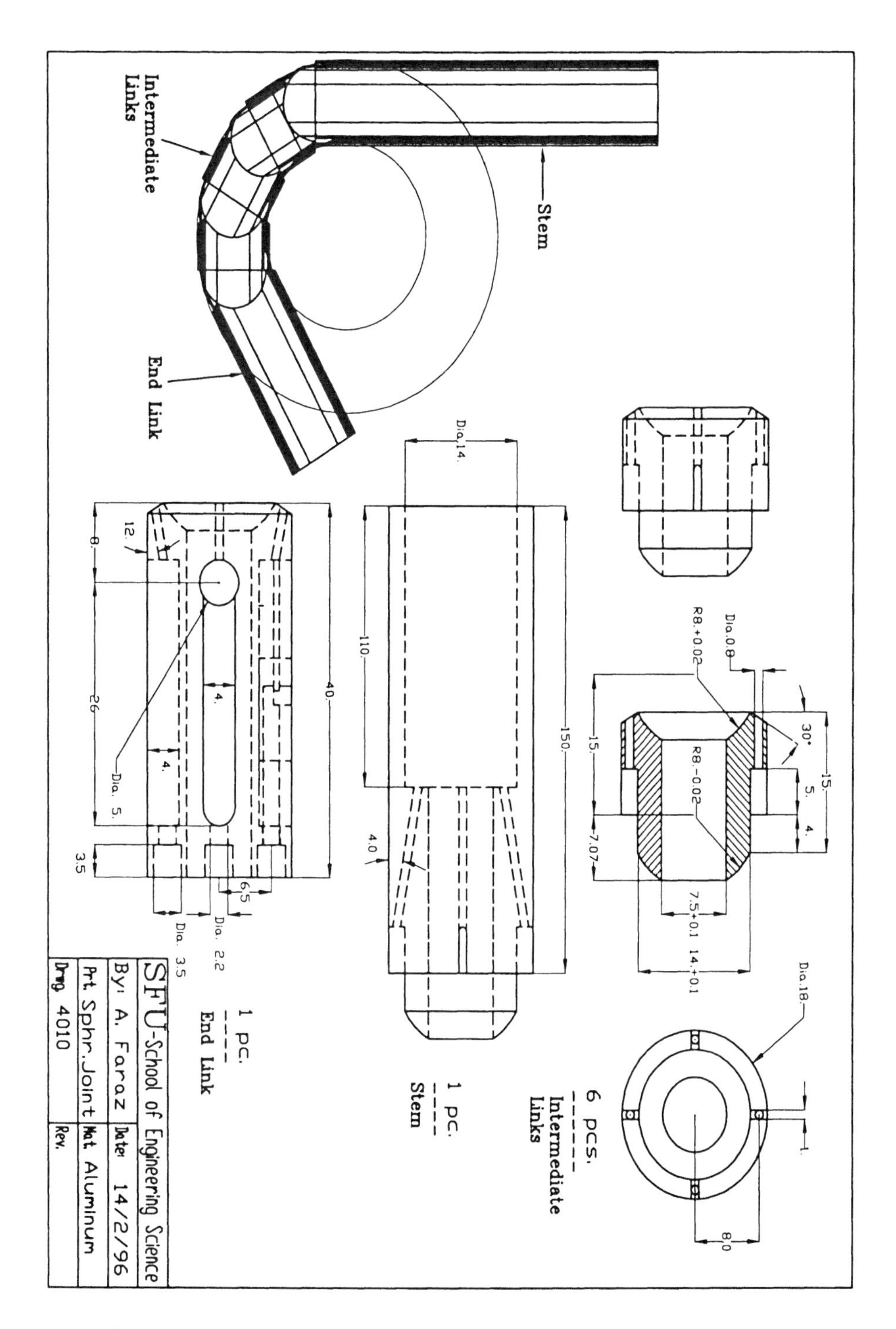

Figure B.3. The multi-spherical joint design actuated by tendon wires.

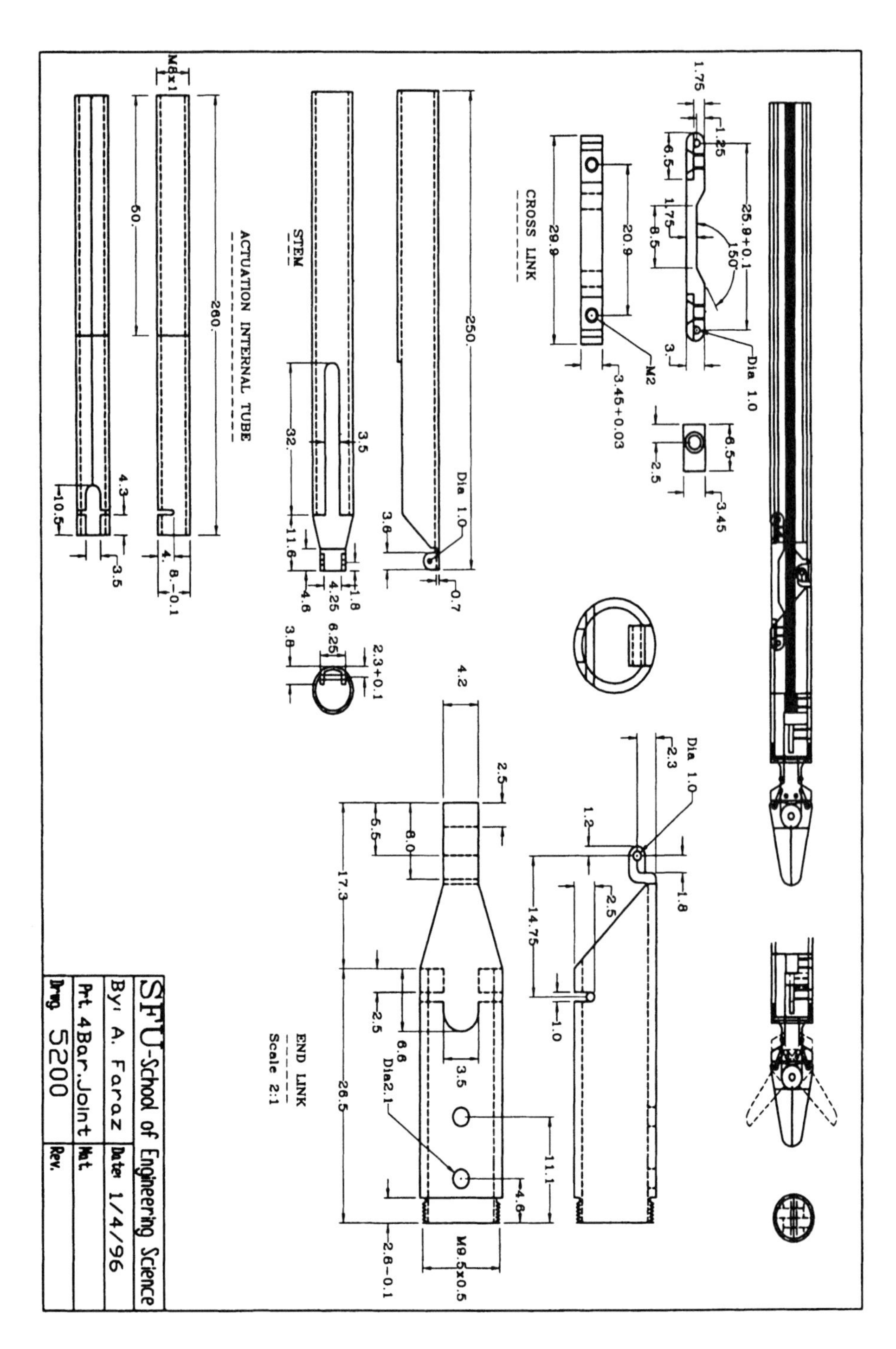

Figure B.4. The design of the grasper head actuated by a flexible shaft.

Appendix C
Jacobian Derivation

Table C.1. The parameters of laparoscopic extender.

Link/Joint	a_i	α_i	d_i	θ_i
1	0	$-90°$	0	θ_1
2	0	$90°$	0	$\theta_2 - 90°$
3	0	0	0	θ_3
4	0	$-90°$	l	0
5	0	$90°$	0	θ_4
6	0	0	l_e	θ_5

The Jacobian of laparoscopic extender (described in Ch.6) with 6 DOF whose coordinates are $[\theta_1, \theta_2, \theta_3, l, \theta_4, \theta_5]^T$ (Fig.C.1) would be a 6×6 matrix. Based on the conventional method of obtaining the Jacobian [78][4], the number of terms in each element of the matrix would become very large, which makes it very difficult to use it in forward or inverse kinematics.

However, there is another Jacobian formulation proposed by Waldron [94] which provides much more compact results. In this method, the fixed frame is located at an intermediate joint instead of its normal location at the base of manipulator, and the Jacobian has the following form:

$$\mathbf{J} = \begin{bmatrix} \mathbf{w}_i \\ \rho_i \times \mathbf{w}_i \end{bmatrix} \tag{C.1}$$

Based on the notation used by Waldron[93] the terms $\mathbf{w}_i$, and ρ_i can be obtained recursively based on the following routine:

$$\begin{aligned} \mathbf{R}_i &= \mathbf{Q}_{i-1}\mathbf{U}_i \\ \mathbf{Q}_i &= \mathbf{R}_i\mathbf{V}_i \\ \mathbf{w}_i &= \mathbf{Q}_{i-1}\mathbf{k} \\ \rho_i &= \rho_{i-1} + \mathbf{R}_{i-1}\mathbf{S}_{i-1} \end{aligned} \tag{C.2}$$

Where $\mathbf{k} = [0, 0, 1]^T$, and the initial conditions are: $\mathbf{Q}_0 = \mathbf{I}, \rho_0 = \mathbf{S}_0 = 0$. The forms for $\mathbf{U}_i$, $\mathbf{V}_i$, and $\mathbf{S}_i$ are:

$$\mathbf{U}_i = \begin{bmatrix} C\theta_i & -S\theta_i & 0 \\ S\theta_i & C\theta_i & 0 \\ 0 & 0 & 1 \end{bmatrix}, \quad \mathbf{V}_i = \begin{bmatrix} 1 & 0 & 0 \\ 0 & C\alpha_i & -S\alpha_i \\ 0 & S\alpha_i & C\alpha_i \end{bmatrix}, \quad \mathbf{S}_i = \begin{bmatrix} a_i \\ 0 \\ r_i \end{bmatrix}$$

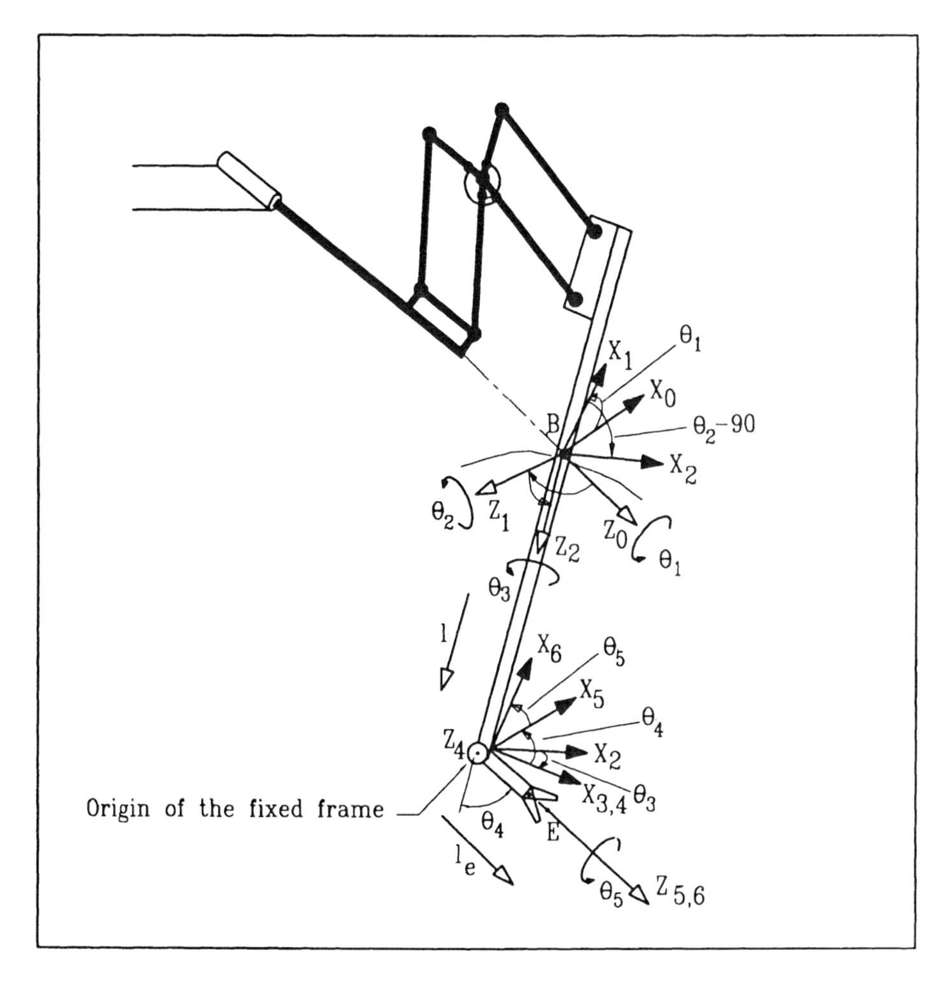

Figure C.1. Joints coordinate frames of the extender and their transformations.

With the reference frame located at Z_4 (Fig.C.1), also having parameters θ_i, α_i, a_i, and r_i as defined in Table C.1 , and working forward in the direction of axis 5, and 6 based on the above recursive routine would provide the following results:

$$\mathbf{w}_5 = \mathbf{k} = \begin{bmatrix} 0 \\ 0 \\ 1 \end{bmatrix}, \rho_5 = \begin{bmatrix} 0 \\ 0 \\ 0 \end{bmatrix}, \rho_5 \times \mathbf{w}_5 = \begin{bmatrix} 0 \\ 0 \\ 0 \end{bmatrix}$$

$$\mathbf{w}_6 = \mathbf{U}_5 \mathbf{V}_5 \mathbf{k} = \begin{bmatrix} C_4 & -S_4 & 0 \\ S_4 & C_4 & 0 \\ 0 & 0 & 1 \end{bmatrix} \begin{bmatrix} 1 & 0 & 0 \\ 0 & 0 & -1 \\ 0 & 1 & 0 \end{bmatrix} \begin{bmatrix} 0 \\ 0 \\ 1 \end{bmatrix} = \begin{bmatrix} S_4 \\ -C_4 \\ 0 \end{bmatrix}$$

$$\rho_6 = \rho_5 + \mathbf{U}_5\mathbf{S}_5 = \begin{bmatrix} 0 \\ 0 \\ 0 \end{bmatrix}$$

$$\rho_6 \times \mathbf{w}_6 = \begin{bmatrix} 0 \\ 0 \\ 0 \end{bmatrix}$$

Now, moving inward along the chain toward axis 3, 2, and 1 we obtain:

$$\mathbf{w}_4 = \mathbf{V}_4^T\mathbf{U}_4^T\mathbf{k} = \begin{bmatrix} 1 & 0 & 0 \\ 0 & 0 & -1 \\ 0 & 1 & 0 \end{bmatrix} \begin{bmatrix} 1 & 0 & 0 \\ 0 & 1 & 0 \\ 0 & 0 & 1 \end{bmatrix} \begin{bmatrix} 0 \\ 0 \\ 1 \end{bmatrix} = \begin{bmatrix} 0 \\ -1 \\ 0 \end{bmatrix}$$

$$\rho_4 = \rho_5 - \mathbf{V}_4^T\mathbf{S}_4 = 0 - \begin{bmatrix} 1 & 0 & 0 \\ 0 & 0 & -1 \\ 0 & 1 & 0 \end{bmatrix} \begin{bmatrix} 0 \\ 0 \\ \ell \end{bmatrix} = \begin{bmatrix} 0 \\ \ell \\ 0 \end{bmatrix}$$

$$\rho_4 \times \mathbf{w}_4 = \begin{bmatrix} 0 \\ \ell \\ 0 \end{bmatrix} \times \begin{bmatrix} 0 \\ -1 \\ 0 \end{bmatrix} = \begin{bmatrix} 0 \\ 0 \\ 0 \end{bmatrix}$$

$$\mathbf{w}_3 = \mathbf{V}_4^T\mathbf{U}_4^T\mathbf{V}_3^T\mathbf{U}_3^T\mathbf{k} = \begin{bmatrix} 1 & 0 & 0 \\ 0 & 0 & -1 \\ 0 & 1 & 0 \end{bmatrix} \begin{bmatrix} C_3 & S_3 & 0 \\ -S_3 & C_3 & 0 \\ 0 & 0 & 1 \end{bmatrix} \begin{bmatrix} 0 \\ 0 \\ 1 \end{bmatrix} = \begin{bmatrix} 0 \\ -1 \\ 0 \end{bmatrix}$$

$$\rho_3 = \rho_4 - \mathbf{V}_4^T\mathbf{U}_4^T\mathbf{V}_3^T\mathbf{S}_3 = \begin{bmatrix} 0 \\ \ell \\ 0 \end{bmatrix} - \begin{bmatrix} 1 & 0 & 0 \\ 0 & 0 & -1 \\ 0 & 1 & 0 \end{bmatrix} \begin{bmatrix} 1 & 0 & 0 \\ 0 & 1 & 0 \\ 0 & 0 & 1 \end{bmatrix} \begin{bmatrix} 0 \\ 0 \\ 0 \end{bmatrix} = \begin{bmatrix} 0 \\ \ell \\ 0 \end{bmatrix}$$

$$\rho_3 \times \mathbf{w}_3 = \begin{bmatrix} 0 \\ \ell \\ 0 \end{bmatrix} \times \begin{bmatrix} 0 \\ -1 \\ 0 \end{bmatrix} = \begin{bmatrix} 0 \\ 0 \\ 0 \end{bmatrix}$$

$$\mathbf{w}_2 = \mathbf{V}_4^T\mathbf{U}_4^T\mathbf{V}_3^T\mathbf{U}_3^T\mathbf{V}_2^T\mathbf{U}_2^T\mathbf{k} =$$

$$\begin{bmatrix} 1 & 0 & 0 \\ 0 & 0 & -1 \\ 0 & 1 & 0 \end{bmatrix} \begin{bmatrix} C_3 & S_3 & 0 \\ -S_3 & C_3 & 0 \\ 0 & 0 & 1 \end{bmatrix} \begin{bmatrix} 1 & 0 & 0 \\ 0 & 0 & 1 \\ 0 & -1 & 0 \end{bmatrix} \begin{bmatrix} S_2 & -C_2 & 0 \\ C_2 & S_2 & 0 \\ 0 & 0 & 1 \end{bmatrix} \begin{bmatrix} 0 \\ 0 \\ 1 \end{bmatrix}$$

$$= \begin{bmatrix} S_3 \\ 0 \\ C_3 \end{bmatrix}$$

$$\rho_2 = \rho_3 - \mathbf{V}_4^T \mathbf{U}_4^T \mathbf{V}_3^T \mathbf{U}_3^T \mathbf{V}_2^T \mathbf{S}_2 = \begin{bmatrix} 0 \\ \ell \\ 0 \end{bmatrix}$$

$$\rho_2 \times \mathbf{w}_2 = \begin{bmatrix} 0 \\ \ell \\ 0 \end{bmatrix} \times \begin{bmatrix} S_3 \\ 0 \\ -C_3 \end{bmatrix} = \begin{bmatrix} \ell C_3 \\ 0 \\ -\ell S_3 \end{bmatrix}$$

$$\mathbf{w}_1 = \mathbf{V}_4^T \mathbf{U}_4^T \mathbf{V}_3^T \mathbf{U}_3^T \mathbf{V}_2^T \mathbf{U}_2^T \mathbf{V}_1^T \mathbf{U}_1^T \mathbf{k} =$$

$$\begin{bmatrix} 1 & 0 & 0 \\ 0 & 0 & -1 \\ 0 & 1 & 0 \end{bmatrix} \begin{bmatrix} C_3 & S_3 & 0 \\ -S_3 & C_3 & 0 \\ 0 & 0 & 1 \end{bmatrix} \begin{bmatrix} 1 & 0 & 0 \\ 0 & 0 & 1 \\ 0 & -1 & 0 \end{bmatrix} \begin{bmatrix} S_2 & -C_2 & 0 \\ C_2 & S_2 & 0 \\ 0 & 0 & 1 \end{bmatrix}$$

$$\begin{bmatrix} 1 & 0 & 0 \\ 0 & 0 & -1 \\ 0 & 1 & 0 \end{bmatrix} \begin{bmatrix} C_1 & S_1 & 0 \\ -S_1 & C_1 & 0 \\ 0 & 0 & 1 \end{bmatrix} \begin{bmatrix} 0 \\ 0 \\ 1 \end{bmatrix} = \begin{bmatrix} C_2 C_3 \\ -S_2 \\ -C_2 S_3 \end{bmatrix}$$

$$\rho_1 = \rho_2 - \mathbf{V}_4^T \mathbf{U}_4^T \mathbf{V}_3^T \mathbf{U}_3^T \mathbf{V}_2^T \mathbf{U}_2^T \mathbf{V}_1^T \mathbf{S}_2 = \begin{bmatrix} 0 \\ \ell \\ 0 \end{bmatrix}$$

$$\rho_1 \times \mathbf{w}_1 = \begin{bmatrix} 0 \\ \ell \\ 0 \end{bmatrix} \times \begin{bmatrix} C_2 C_3 \\ -S_2 \\ -C_2 S_3 \end{bmatrix} = \begin{bmatrix} -\ell C_2 S_3 \\ 0 \\ -\ell C_2 C_3 \end{bmatrix}$$

Therefore the final Jacobian after assembling all $\mathbf{w}_i$ and $\rho_i \times \mathbf{w}_i$ elements in the form of 6×6 matrix would be :

$$\mathbf{J} = \begin{bmatrix} \mathbf{w}_i \\ \rho_i \times \mathbf{w}_i \end{bmatrix} = \begin{bmatrix} C_2 C_3 & S_3 & 0 & 0 & 0 & S_4 \\ -S_2 & 0 & -1 & 0 & 0 & -C4 \\ -C_2 S_3 & C_3 & 0 & 0 & 1 & 0 \\ -lC_2 S_3 & lC_3 & 0 & 0 & 0 & 0 \\ 0 & 0 & 0 & -1 & 0 & 0 \\ -lC_2 C_3 & -lS_3 & 0 & 0 & 0 & 0 \end{bmatrix} \qquad \text{(C.3)}$$

References

[1] S. Payandeh A. Faraz and Andon Salvarinov. Design of force reflecting grasper through stiffness modulation for endosurgry: Theory and experiments. In *The International Journal of Mechatronics*. Pergamon Press, To be published in 2000.

[2] Andronic Devices Ltd., Suite 140-13120 Vanier Place, Richmond, B.C. V6V 2J2. *Endex, Endoscopy Positioning System, Product Catalogue*, 1993.

[3] Armstrong Projects Ltd., Beaconsfield, UK. *Products Catalogue*, 1995.

[4] H. Asada and J.-J. E. Slotine. *Robot Analysis and Control.* John Wiley and Sons, MIT, 1986.

[5] R. W. Bailey and J. L. Flowers. *Complications of Laparoscopic Surgery*, chapter 1, pages 3–4. Quality Medical Publishing Inc., 1995.

[6] T. Baumeister, E. A. Avallone, and T. Baumeister III. *Mark's Standard Handbook for Mechanical Engineers.* McGraw-Hill, 8th edition, 1978. pages 5.51-52, 5.5, 6.67-68.

[7] T. Baumeister, E. A. Avallone, and T. Bauumeister III. *Mark's Standard Handbook for Mechanical Engineers,*. Mc Graw-Hill, 8th edition, 1978. page 3.26.

[8] M. C. Becquet. *Teleoperation: Numerical Simulation and Experimental Validation.* 1992. Pages 139-161.

[9] Belt Technologies Inc., 11 Bowles Road, P.O. Box 468, Agawam, Ma 01001-0468, U.S.A. *Design Guide and Engineers Reference for Metal Belts*, 1996.

[10] H. R. Beurrier. Surgical suturing device. In U.S. *Patent Number : 5,308,353*, May 1994.

[11] R. G. Budynas. *Advanced Strength and Applied Stress Analysis.* McGraw-Hill, 1977. pages 151-160.

[12] P. F. Byrd and M. D. Friedman. *Handbook of Elliptic Integrals for Engineers and Scientists.* Springer - Verlag, 2nd edition, 1971. pages 10,12,39,299-301.

[13] C. G. L. Cao. A task analysis laparoscopic surgery: Requirements for remote manipulation and endoscopic tool design. Master's thesis, Simon Fraser University, School of Kinesiology, April 1996. pages 36-69.

[14] Computer Motion Inc., 130 Cremona Dr., Goleta, CA 93117, U.S.A. *AESOP : Automated Endoscopic System for Optimal Positioning*, 1994.

[15] A. Damon, H. W. Stoudt, and R. A. McFarland. *The Human Body in Equipment Design.* Harvard University Press, 1966. pages 221-223.

[16] J. Dargahi, M. Parameswaran, and S. Payandeh. A micromachined piezoelectric tactile sensor for use in endoscopic graspers. In *Proceedings of International Conference on Intelligent Robots and Systems*, pages 566–579. IEEE, October 98.

[17] A. De and U. Tasch. Modulating the end-point compliance of a two-dof manipulator to its full rank: Theory and hardware implementation. In *ASME, DSC-Vol. 55-1*, pages 193–198, 1994.

[18] C.W. deSilva. *Control Sensors and Actuators*, chapter 2, page 53. Prentice Hall, 1989.

[19] A. D. Deutschman, W. J. Michels, and C. E. Wilson. *Machine Design, Theory and Practice.* Macmillan, 1975. pages 663-664.

[20] K. Doel and D. Pai. Performance measures for robot manipulators: A unified approach. In *The International Journal of Robotics Research*, volume 15, pages 92–111. MIT, February 1996.

[21] Ethicon, Johnson and Johnson. *Endo-Surgery, Product catalogue and price list*, 1993.

[22] A. Faraz and S. Payandeh. Design and analysis of tunable springs in haptic interface of endoscopic graspers. In *Sixth Annual Symposium*

on Haptic Interfaces for Virtual Environment and Teleoperator Systems, pages 69–76. ASME, International Mechaniccal Engineering Congress and Exxposition, Dallas, Texas, November 1997.

[23] A. Faraz and S. Payandeh. A robotics case study: Optimal design for laparoscopic stands. In *Proceedings of IEEE International conference on Robotics and Automation(ICRA'97)*, volume 2, pages 1553–1560, April 1997.

[24] A. Faraz and S. Payandeh. Suturing device. In U.S. *patent Number: 5,766,186.* Simon Fraser University, 1997.

[25] A. Faraz and S. Payandeh. Synthesis and workspace study of endoscopic extenders with flexible stem. In *Journal of Mechanical Design*, volume 119, pages 412–414, September 1997.

[26] A. Faraz and S. Payandeh. Adjustable surgical stand. In U.S. *Patent Number. 5,824,007.* Simon Fraser University, 1998.

[27] A. Faraz and S. Payandeh. Force reflecting grasper. In *US Patent Application.* Simon Fraser University, 1998.

[28] A. Faraz and S. Payandeh. A robotic case study: Optimal design for laparoscopic positioning stand. In *The International Journal of Robotics Research*, volume 17, pages 986–995, September 1998.

[29] A. Faraz and S. Payandeh. Application of robotics in endoscopic surgery. In *Proc. 15th Canadian Congress of Applied Mechanics*, volume 1, pages 252–253, May ,28,1995.

[30] A. Faraz and S. Payandeh. The frictional moment in spherical joints. In *Proceedings 15th Canadian Congress of Applied Mechanics*, volume 2, May ,29,1995. pages 820-821.

[31] A. Faraz and S. Payandeh. Kinematic modelling and trajectory planning for tele-laparoscopic manipulating system. In *Robotica*, To be published in 2000.

[32] A. Faraz, S. Payandeh, and A. Nagy. Issues and design concepts in endoscopic extenders. In *Proceedings of 6th International Federation of Automatic Control Symposium(IFAC-MMS)*, pages 109–114, MIT, June 1995.

[33] A. Faraz, S. Payandeh, and A. Salvarinov. Design of haptic interface through stiffness modulation for endosurgery: Theory and experiments. In *Proc. of IEEE, International Conference on Robotics and Automation*, pages 1007–1013, May 1998.

[34] P. A. Finlay and M. H. Ornstein. Controlling the movement of a surgical laparoscope. In *Engineering in Medicine and Biology Magazine*, volume 14(3). IEEE, May 1995. pages 289-291.

[35] H. Fischer, B. Neisius, and R. Trapp. Tactile feedback for endoscopic surgery. In *Interactive Technology and the New Paradim for Healthcare*, pages 114–117. IOS Press and Ohmsha, 1995.

[36] C. T. Frantzides. *Laparoscopic and Thoracoscopic Surgery*, pages 2–5. Mosby, 1995.

[37] J. Funda, B. Eldridge, K. Gruben, S. Gomory, and R. Taylor. Comparison of two manipulator designs for laparoscopic surgery. In *Telemanipulator and Telepresence Technologies, SPIE*, volume 2351, pages 172–183, 1994.

[38] C. Gosselin and J. Angeles. A global performance index for the kinematic optimization of robotic manipulators. In *Journal of Mechanical Design*, volume 113, pages 220–226. ASME, September 1991.

[39] P. S. Green, J. W. Hill, and A. Shah. Telepresence surgery. In *Engineering in Medicine and Biology Magazine*, volume 14, pages 324–329. IEEE, May 1995.

[40] V. Gupta, N. P. Reddy, and P. Batur. Forces in surgical tools: Comparison between laparoscopic and surgical forceps. In *IEEE, Engineering in Medicine and Biology, Paper No. 668*, 1996.

[41] V. Gupta, N. P. Reddy, and P. Batur. Forces in laparoscopic surgical tools. In *Presence*, volume 6, pages 218–228, April 1997.

[42] L. J. Gutkowski and G. L. Kinzel. A coulomb friction model for spherical joints. In *ASME, DE-Vol. 45*, pages 243–250, 1992.

[43] G. J. Hamlin and A.C. Sanderson. A novel concentric multi-link spherical joint with parallel robotics applications. In *IEEE Proc.*, pages 1267–1272, 1995.

[44] R. Heimberger. Flexible endoscope. In U.S. *Patent Number: 5,349,942*, Richard Wolf GmbH, September 1994.

[45] J. W. Hill, P. S. Green, J. F. Jensen, Y. Gosfu, and A. S. Shah. Telepresence surgery demonstration system. In *Proc. IEEE, 1050-4729/94*, pages 2302–2307, 1994.

[46] I. Imam, M. Skreiner, and J. P. Sadler. A new solution to coulomb friction in mechanism bearings: Theory and application. In *Trans. ASME*, volume 103, pages 764–775, 1981.

[47] T. Ivergard. *Handbook of Control Room Design and Ergonomics.* Taylor and Francis, 1989. pages 117-125.

[48] B. G. Jackson and L. B. Rosenberg. Force feedback and medical simulation. In *Interactive Technology and the New Paradigm for Healthcare*, pages 1476–1481. IOS Press and Ohmsha, 1995.

[49] J. Jensen. Remote center positioner. In *World Intellectual Property Organization*, volume WO 94/26167. SRI International, November 1994.

[50] A. K. Klein and T. A. Miklos. Spatial robotic isotropy. In *The International Journal of Robotics Research*, volume 10, pages 426–437, 1991.

[51] K. F. Laurin-Kovitz, J. E. Colgate, and S. D. R. Carnes. Design of components for programmable passive impedance. In *IEEE, Int. Conf. on Robotics and Automation, Sacramento, Ca.*, pages 1476–1481, 1991.

[52] Laurus Medical Group, 30 Hughes Suite 202, Irvine, CA 92718. *The Laurus PC Suturing System, Product Catalogue*, 1995.

[53] M. Y. Lee, A. G. Erdman, and Y. Gutman. Development of kinematic/ kinetic performance tools in synthesis of multi-dof mechanisms. In *Journal of Mechanical Design*, volume 115, pages 462–472. ASME, September Sept.1993.

[54] C. Lipson and R. Juvinall. *Handbook of Stress and Strength.* Macmillan, 1963. Ch.7, pages 81-88.

[55] I. M. C. Macintyre. *Practical Laparoscopy Surgery*, chapter 4, pages 26–27. Butterworth-Heinemann Ltd., 1994.

[56] T. Matsumaru. U.S. patent number: 5,174,277. In *Endoscope*, Kabushiki Kaisha Toshiba, Kawasaki, Japan, 1994.

[57] D. G. Matsuura and C. Boyll. Deflecting endoscope. In U.S. *Patent Number: 5,307,803*, Intramed Laboratories, San Diego, Calif., U.S.A., May 1994.

[58] A. Melzer. Intelligent surgical instrument system ISIS. In *Endoscopic Surgery and Allied Technologies*, volume 1, pages 165–170, 1993.

[59] A. Melzer, M. O. Schurr, M. M. Lirici, B. Klemm, D. Stockel, and G. Buess. Future trends in endoscopic suturing. In *Endoscopic Surgery and Allied Technologies*, volume 2, pages 78–82, 1994.

[60] T. N. Mitchell, J. Robertson, A. G. Nagy, and A. Lomax. Three-dimensional endoscopic imaging for minimal access surgery. In *J.R. Coll. Surg. Edinb.*, volume 38, pages 285–292, 1993.

[61] S. Mittal, U. Tasch, and Y. Wang. A redundant actuation scheme for independent modulations of stiffness and position of a robotic joint: Design, implementation and experimental evaluation. In *ASME, DSC-Vol. 49, Advances in Robotics, Mechatronics, and Haptic Interfaces*, pages 247–256, 1993.

[62] A. Nagy. Head of Laparoscopic Surgery, Department of Surgery, University of British Columbia, and Vancouver General Hospital, 1995. Personal Communications.

[63] A.G. Nagy and S. Payandeh. Endoscopic end-effectors. In *The National Design Engineering Conference*, volume 94-DE-5. ASME, March 1994.

[64] B. Neisius, P. Dautzenberg, and R.Trapp. Robotic manipulator for endoscopic handling of surgical effectors and cameras. In *First International Symposium on Medical Robotics and Computer Assisted Surgery (MRCAS)*, pages 1–7, July 1994.

[65] F. C. Park and R. W. Brockett. Kinematic dexterity of robotic mechanisms. In *The International Journal of Robotics Research*, volume 13, pages 1–15, 1994.

[66] M. Patkin and L. Isabel. Ergonomics, engineering and surgery of endosurgical dissection. In *J.R. Coll. Surg. Edinb.*, volume 40, pages 120–132, April 1995.

[67] S. Payandeh. Force propagation models in laparoscopic tools and trainers. In *Proceedings of International Conference on Engineering in Medicine and Biology.* IEEE, May 97. Paper number 531.

[68] J. Perissat, A. Cuschieri, G. Buess, and J. perissat. *Laparoscopic Cholecystectomy.* Operative Manual of Endoscopic Surgery, Springer-Verlag, 1992. Pages209-232.

[69] S. Pheasant. *Bodyspace, Anthropometry, Ergonomics and the Design of Work.* Taylor and Francis, 2nd edition, 1996. Pages 93-97.

[70] J. P. Piene, D. A. Kontarinis, and R.D. Howe. A tactile sensing and display system for surgical applications. In *Interactive Technology and the New Paradigm for Healthcare*, pages 283–288. IOS Press and Ohmsha, 1995.

[71] H. H. Rininsland. Basics of robotics and manipulators in endoscopic surgery. In *Endoscopic Surgery and Allied Technologies*, volume 1, pages 154–159, 1993.

[72] T. Sakaki and S. Tachi. Impedance controlled master-slave manipulation system. In *Journak of Advance Robotics*, volume 7, pages 3–24, 1993.

[73] J. K. Salisbury and J. J. Craig. Articulated hands: Force control and kinematic issues. In *International Journal of Robotics Research*, volume 1, pages 4–17, 1982.

[74] Sava Industries Inc., 4 North Corporate Dr., P.O. Box 30, Riverdale, New Jersey 07457-0030, U.S.A. *Flexible Push-pull Shafts and Cables*, 1997.

[75] A. Senagore. *General Techniques of Laparoscopic Surgery*. Butterworth, 1994. Ch.10, pages 107-113.

[76] T. B. Sheridan. *Telerobotics, Automation, and Human Supervisory Control*. MIT Press, Cambridge, MA., 1992.

[77] Y. J. Shin and C. H. Kim. An analytical solution for spherical joint mechanism including coulomb friction. In *6th International Pacific Conference on Automotive Engineering*, pages 383–389, 1991.

[78] M. W. Spong and M. Vidyasagar. *Robot Dynamics and Control*. John Wiley and Sons, 1989.

[79] Stock Drive Products. *Handbook of Timing Belts, Chains and Friction Drives, Catalog D210*, 1991.

[80] Storz. *General catalogue of endoscopic instruments*. Karl Storz-Endoskope, 1992.

[81] R.H. Sturges and S. Laowattana. A flexible, tendon-controlled device for endoscopy. In *International Journal of Robotics Research*, volume 12(2), pages 121–131, 1993.

[82] S. M. Sukthankar and N. P. Reddy. Toward force feedback in laparoscopic surgical tools. In *Engineering in Medicine & Biology*. IEEE, 1994. Paper No. 479.

[83] S. M. Sukthankar and N. P. Reddy. Force feedback issues in minimally invasive surgery. In *Interactive Technology and the New Paradim for Healthcare*, pages 375–379. IOS Press and Ohmsha, 1995.

[84] Surgical Innovations Ltd., Clayton Park, Clayton Wood Rise, Leeds, LS16 6RF, UK. *Products Catalogue*, 1995.

[85] Z. Szabo, J. Hunter, G. Berci, J. Sackier, and A. Cuschieri. Analysis of surgical movements during suturing in laparoscopy. In *Endoscopy Surgery*, volume 2, pages 55–61, 1994.

[86] R. H. Taylor, J. Funda, B. Edridge, S. Gomory, K. Gruben, D. LaRose, M. Talamini, L. Kavoussi, and J. Anderson. A telerobotic assistant for laparoscopic surgery. In *Engineering in Medicine and Biology Magazine*, volume 14, pages 279–288. IEEE, May 1995.

[87] F. Tendick, R. W. Jennings, G. Thrap, and L. Stark. Sensing and manipulation problems in endoscopic surgery: Experiment, analysis, and observation. In *Presence*, volume 2, pages 66–81. MIT, Winter 1993.

[88] V. Van Hemert tot Dingshof, M. Lazeroms, A. Van der Ham, W. Jongkind, and G. Honderd. Force reflection for a laparoscopic forceps. In *IEEE Engineering in Medicine and Biology*, 1996. Paper Number 118.

[89] H. S. Tzou and Y. Rong. Contact dynamics of a spherical joint and a jointed truss-cell system. In *American Institute of Aeronautics Astronautics Journal*, volume 29(1), pages 81–88, 1991.

[90] K. Uchino. *Piezoelectric Actuators and Ultrasonic motors*, chapter 3. Kluwer Academic Publishers, 1997.

[91] U.S. Surgical. *Product catalogue, Auto-Suture*, 1996.

[92] J. Vertute and P. Coiffet. *Teleoperation and Robotics, Evolution and Development*, volume 3A. Kogan Page, 1985. Page 23.

[93] K. J. Waldron. Geometrically based manipulator rate control algorithms. In *Mechanism and Machine theory*, volume 17, pages 379–385, 1982.

[94] K. J. Waldron and S. J. Bolin S. L. Wang. A study of the Jacobian matrix of serial manipulators. In *Transactions of ASME*, volume 107, pages 230–238, June 1985.

[95] J. M. Wendlandt and S. S. Sastry. Design and control of a simplified Stewart platform for endoscopy. In *Conference on Decision and Control*, pages 357–362. IEEE, December 1994.

[96] D. E. Whitney. Resolved motion rate control of manipulators and human prostheses. In *IEEE Trans. Man-Machine Systems*, volume 10, 1969.

[97] Y. Yokokohji and T. Yoshikawa. Bilateral control of master-slave manipulators for ideal kinesthetic coupling. In *IEEE, Int. Workshop on Intelligent Robots and Systems (IROS 90)*, pages 355–362, 1990.

[98] T. Yoshikawa. Manipulability of robotic mechanisms. In *International Journal of Robotic Research*, volume 4, pages 3–9. MIT, Summer 1985.

About the Authors

Ali Faraz was born in Iran on 1958. Received his BS from University of Southern California(1980) in mechanical engineering, and MS in manufacturing from University of Manchester(1986). He has been working in industry for over 12 years and his interest for the design of surgical tools and medical robotics got him involved in continuing with his Ph.D. research. His research and development at the Experimental Robotics Laboratory (ERL) in the faculty of Engineering Science of Simon Fraser University) led to several new surgical prototype developments, 2 U.S.patents, and over 12 publications. This book is the result of this research and its content is based on his Ph.D. thesis. His general interests is mechanical design, kinematic synthesis and optimization. Currently he is working with Creo Products Inc. in British Columbia, Canada as analyst and mechanical designer.

Shahram Payandeh was born in Iran on 1957. Received his BS and MS degrees from University of Akron (Ohio) and his Ph.D. degree from University of Toronto (Canada) all in Mechanical Engineering. His field of research has been in the area of robotics. His focus is in the design and control of special purpose mechanisms such as robotic devices. He has more than 90 technical publications in these areas and a number of patents. The work of this book is based on his proposal to investigate potential mechanical and robotic designs of devices which can help the surgeon during Minimally Invasive Surgical procedures. He is currently an Associate Professor at the School of Engineering Science of Simon Fraser University in Burnaby, British Columbia, Canada.

Index

CPSIA information can be obtained at www.ICGtesting.com
Printed in the USA
LVOW012127301111

257292LV00006B/22/A

9 780792 377924